DATE DUE

JUL 7 1986		
Aug 5 SEP 09 1994		

DEMCO 38-297

Cutaneous Laser Therapy:
Principles and Methods

Cutaneous Laser Therapy: Principles and Methods

edited by

K. A. ARNDT
J. M. NOE
S. ROSEN

Beth Israel Hospital and Harvard Medical School, Boston, Massachusetts.

A Wiley Medical Publication

JOHN WILEY & SONS
Chichester . New York . Brisbane . Toronto . Singapore

Library of Congress Cataloging in Publication Data:
Main entry under title:

Cutaneous laser therapy; principles and methods

(A Wiley medical publication)
Based on papers presented at a symposium sponsored by
the Laser Unit, Beth Israel Hospital, Boston and
the Dept. of Continuing Education. Harvard Medical
School, in Sept. 1981
  Includes bibliographical references and index.
  1. Lasers—Therapeutic use—Congresses.
  2. Skin—Diseases—Treatment—Congresses.
  I. Arndt, Kenneth A.   II. Noe, Joel M.
  III. Rosen, S. (Seymour)
  IV. Beth Israel Hospital (Boston, Mass.). Laser Unit.

V. Harvard Medical School. Dept. of Continuing Education.
RL120.L37C87   1983   616.5'0631   82–17379

ISBN 0 471 90075 3 (U.S.)

British Library Cataloguing in Publication Data:

Cutaneous laser therapy: principles and methods
  1. Skin—Diseases   2. Lasers in medicine
  I. Arndt, K. A.   II. Noe, J. M.
  III. Rosen, S.
  616.5'065   RL71

ISBN 0 471 90075 3

Typeset by Activity, Salisbury and printed in
Great Britain by Page Bros. (Norwich) Ltd.

We would like to dedicate this book to our families for their love and support

Contributors

R. Rox Anderson BS
  Physicist, Department of Dermatology, Massachusetts General Hospital, Boston

Kenneth A. Arndt, MD
  Chief, Department of Dermatology and Co-Chairman, Laser Unit, Beth Israel Hospital; Associate Professor of Dermatology, Harvard Medical School, Boston

Philip L. Bailin, MD
  Chairman, Department of Dermatology, Cleveland Clinic Foundation, Cleveland

Donna B. C. Bourgelais, BS
  Director, Research and Development, Laakmann Electro-Optics, Inc., San Juan Capistrano, California

John A. Dixon, MD
  Professor of Surgery, Adjunct Professor of Medicine, and Director, Endoscopic and Laser Surgery Unit, University of Utah Medical Center, Salt Lake City

James L. Finley, MD
  Fellow in Pathology, Beth Israel Hospital, and Clinical Fellow in Pathology, Harvard Medical School, Boston

Barbara A. Gilchrest, MD
  Associate Dermatologist, Beth Israel Hospital; Assistant Professor of Dermatology, Harvard Medical School, Boston

Leon Goldman, MD
  Professor Emeritus of Dermatology, Former Director Laser Laboratory,

University of Cincinnati Medical Center; Director, Laser Research Laboratory and Director, Laser Treatment Center, The Jewish Hospital, Cincinnati

ROBERT M. GOLDWYN, MD
Head of the Division of Plastic Surgery, Beth Israel Hospital; Clinical Professor of Surgery, Harvard Medical School, Boston

IRVING ITZKAN, PH.D.
Chairman, Optics Committee, AVCO Everett Research Laboratory, Inc., Everett

S. MICHAEL KALICK, PhD
Assistant in Psychiatry, Beth Israel Hospital; Instructor of Psychology, Harvard Medical School, Assistant Professor of Psychology, University of Massachusetts, Boston

JOEL M. NOE, MD
Co-Chairman, Laser Unit, Beth Israel Hospital; Assistant Clinical Professor of Surgery (Plastic Surgery), Harvard Medical School, Boston

JOHN A. PARRISH, MD
Department of Dermatology, Massachusetts General Hospital; Associate Professor of Dermatology, Harvard Medical School, Boston

SEYMOUR ROSEN, MD
Associate Pathologist and Director, Surgical Pathology, and Co-Chairman, Laser Unit, Beth Israel Hospital; Associate Professor of Pathology, Harvard Medical School, Boston

ROBERT S. STERN, MD
Associate Dermatologist, Beth Israel Hospital; Assistant Professor of Dermatology, Harvard Medical School, Boston

STEPHEN TANG, MD
Laser Unit, Beth Israel Hospital, Boston

SAN WAN, MD, PHD
Clinical and Research Fellow in Dermatology, Massachusetts General Hospital, Boston

Contents

Introduction
K. A. Arndt, J. M. Noe, and S. Rosen

SECTION I HISTORICAL PERSPECTIVES

SECTION II INTERACTION OF LASERS WITH THE SKIN

SECTION III PORT WINE STAINS

SECTION IV TREATMENT OF CUTANEOUS LESIONS OTHER THAN PORT WINE STAINS

SECTION V PSYCHOSOCIAL ASPECTS OF FACIAL DISFIGUREMENT AND THE EFFECTS OF MODIFICATION VIA LASER THERAPY

SECTION VI THE FUTURE OF LASERS IN MEDICINE

Introduction

During the last 20 years, lasers have become increasingly accepted as instruments of great usefulness for dermatologic therapy and photobiologic investigation. The intense laser radiation is able to alter a variety of cutaneous tissues by thermal injury in either a nonspecific but highly controlled manner or with a high degree of specificity. The optical characteristics of skin may make possible the intriguing goal of treating specific intracutaneous targets with radiation that passes intact through unaffected and unaltered viable cutaneous tissue [1].

Three forces have served to stimulate interest in the development of lasers in dermatology and plastic surgery. First was the fact that the skin had numerous excellent qualities as a test model for the study of the effects of lasers on humans [2]. It was accessible, it proved to be safe for short- and long-term laser exposure, and it provided a tissue available for controlled investigation which also was affected by diseases for which lasers provided a potential clinical application. The second force was that of the work of Dr. Leon Goldman, who saw the skin as a model for studying these effects and sought to show the distinct qualities and advantages of lasers relative to other modalities of treatment [3,4], and the work of Drs. Harvey Lash, Morton Maser, and David Apfelberg and their colleagues at the Palo Alto Medical Clinic, who demonstrated the effectiveness of the argon laser [4]. The third factor was investigative work carried out by ophthalmologists [5,6].

The first laser developed, the ruby laser, gained acceptance for photocoagulation of retinal detachments. As argon lasers became available, they proved even more effective for ophthalmologic use as well as for treatment of vascular lesions of the skin. The blue-green light from the argon laser was thought to be specifically absorbed by intraluminal red blood cells, leading to thermal damage, thrombosis, and lightening of the color of vascular lesions. As time has passed, the relative specificity of the argon laser–hemoglobin interaction has been questioned and the precise mode of inducing improvement in clinical lesions has become a subject of ongoing research [7].

Ruby and argon lasers have been used primarily for their effects on vascular lesions, but they also have been utilized because of their absorption by pigments such as melanin and that in traumatic or decorative tattoos. The other laser that has been found most useful in laser medicine has been the carbon dioxide (CO_2) laser. This instrument not only can vaporize tissue but can cut, as would a scalpel, resulting in many potentially unique applications. Many other lasers exist and at least 12 systems have been used in biomedical investigations or on cutaneous structures, but the argon and CO_2 appear to be the most clinically adaptable and effective lasers at this time.

The unique properties of lasers create an enormous potential for *specific* therapy of a variety of diseases of the skin [8]. Within the next few years, it should be possible to define the tissue reflectance characteristics of lesions with spectrophotometers and then choose a wavelength for laser phototherapy that will maximize lesion absorption and minimize other epidermal or dermal damage. Before this can happen, however, we need much more information about the pathophysiologic response of tissues to laser radiation and about optimal laser techniques. Precise and sophisticated photobiologic and clinical–pathologic studies will allow progress in this expanding and exciting field.

Interest in lasers and skin has been increasing rapidly over the past few years. The medical literature concerning the clinical effects of lasers on skin has progressed from descriptive and anecdotal reports to prospective, histologically controlled studies. Many articles describing basic laser photochemistry and the theoretical aspects of laser and skin optics and their potential application to clinical medicine have been published. Laser medicine has begun to 'come of age'.

This volume is meant to put the large amount of recent data about lasers and skin into a critical perspective defining principles in concert with pragmatic issues of technique. Much of the information was originally presented at a symposium 'Cutaneous Laser Therapy' sponsored by the Laser Unit, Beth Israel Hospital, Boston, and the Department of Continuing Education, Harvard Medical School, in September, 1981. The Beth Israel Hospital Laser Unit is a group consisting of basic scientists, physicians, nurses, and psychologists. Our studies, which have particularly reflected the fruitful collaboration of dermatologists, plastic surgeons, and pathologists, have been aided by support from Coherent Laboratories, Inc. and grants from the American Society of Aesthetic Surgery and the Education Foundation of the Society for Plastic and Reconstructive Surgery.

KENNETH A. ARNDT
JOEL M. NOE
SEYMOUR ROSEN

References

1. Arndt K. A., Noe, J. M. Lasers in dermatology. *Arch Dermatol.* 1982; **118**: 293–5.
2. Goldman, L. Effects of new laser systems on the skin. *Arch. Dermatol.* 1973; **108**:385–90.
3. Goldman, L., Rockwell, R. J. Jr. Laser reaction in living tissue. In: *Lasers in Medicine.* New York: Gordon and Breach, 1972:163–85.
4. Apfelberg, D. B., Maser, M. R., Lash, H. Argon laser management of cutaneous vascular deformities. A preliminary report. *West J. Med.* 1976; **124**:99–101.
5. Zweng, K. M., Flocks, M. Clinical experiences with laser photocoagulation. *Fedn. Proc.* 1965; **24**:565–70.
6. Zinn, K. M. Clinical aspects of ophthalmic argon lasers. *Lasers in Surgery and Medicine.* 1981; **1**:289–322.
7. van Gemert, M. J. C., Hulsbergen-Henning, J. P. A model approach to laser coagulation of dermal vascular lesions. *Arch Dermatol.* 1981; **270**:429–39.
8. Anderson, R. R., Parrish, J. A. Microvasculature can be selectively damaged by dye lasers: a basic theory and experimental evidence in human skin. *Lasers in Surgery and Medicine.* 1981; **1**:263–76.

SECTION I
Historical Perspectives

Cutaneous Laser Therapy: Principles and Methods
Edited by K. A. Arndt, J. M. Noe, and S. Rosen
© 1983 John Wiley & Sons Ltd

1

Historical Perspective: Personal Reflections

Leon Goldman

Lasers are an important part of the renaissance of photobiology, photodiagnostics, and phototherapy in dermatology. The laser was conceived in 1917, when Einstein wrote *Zur Quantum Theorie der Strahlung* [1]. He established the concepts of stimulated emission, stimulated absorption, and spontaneous emission. Studies on microwave amplification by Basov and Prokhorov in Russia, and Townes and Weber in the United States, furthered these concepts and extended lasers into the optical frequency range suggested by Schawlow and Townes in 1958, and, according to current controversy, also by Gould. On July 7, 1960, T. H. Maiman of Hughes Aircraft Research Laboratories operated the first laser—the brilliant coherent red light of a ruby laser at 694.4 nm. New lasers developed rapidly after this and continue to be developed now for use in laser medicine.

3

Early clinical use

The first medical application of lasers was for the treatment of retinal detachment. This was done by focusing ruby laser impacts about the retinal detachment to 'weld' it to the adjacent tissue. At about the same time, the ruby laser was also used to vaporize chronic hemorrhage in the eye and to try to arrest hemorrhage from bleeding vessels. After the initial retinal laser surgery, cutaneous laser therapy was started. In the early days, it was often difficult to get the laser off the optical bench so it would be more flexible for clinical use. It was difficult also, with limited budgets, to buy, rather than to borrow, an expensive laser instrument with investigative clinical use potential. Our physicists and engineers would modify the instruments with regard to single mode, flexibility, and sterilizability. Initially, various optical instruments such as mirrors, prisms, gimbal mounts, etc. were used to carry the beam from the bench to the lesion of the animal or patient. The laser operating room at the National Cancer Institute also had difficulties with transmission of the laser beam from the point of origin through various crude optical fibers to the operating table. This resulted in inadequate laser treatment, and consequently poor and discouraging results.

One difficulty we encountered in clinical experiments was choosing the appropriate type of controls for the development of thermocoagulation necrosis. The high-frequency electrosurgical unit was one type, but the problem was to equate energy and power densities. The comparison often was made by the degree of clinical reaction. The other controls for laser surgery have been the scalpel, cryosurgery, electrocautery, and now, high-output incoherent infrared radiation. The latter is being used especialy in Germany in the operating room for hemostasis and for the treatment of hemorrhoids (G. Nath, personal communication).

Safety

Shortly after the discovery of the ruby laser, there developed concern about the hazards of lasers to the eyes and the skin. The early studies on eye safety were done with the ruby laser, 20 J/cm^2, on the eyes of rabbits and monkeys. The early studies on safety for the skin were done on human skin. Exposure of the human skin to the ruby laser showed a nonspecific thermocoagulation necrosis similar to that of electric burns. Occasional dysplastic cells were found in the epidermis. Studies of chronic ruby laser radiation, 20 J/cm^2 exposures, on normal skin and on precancerous spots showed no carcinogenic effects [2].

As each new laser system was introduced, there was interest first in the development and use of laser safety programs, and then on its possible medical applications. The laser was first reviewed in detail with a laser physicist and then safety programs were outlined with eye experiments in animals and on the skin in humans. Initially, it was difficult to convince the laser industry to develop adequate laser safety programs. It became necessary to learn something about the photobiology of the particular laser under study. Laser safety programs have continued with regard to: first, safety of the laser itself, in its manufacture and operation; second, laser safety programs for the patient and for the operator; and third, the laser's effect on environmental pollution. For laser manufacture and testing it became clear that workers should have eye protection and protection from high-output electrical systems. The potential risks are great—in our program for the development of the Q-switched laser for the treatment of tattoos there was one fatality in a plant accident. In the United States it is now the custom for an instrument to be certified with a safety mark and the exit area specifically marked. Protection of the patient relates to eye protection, skin protection, and protection from flammability of drapes in the operating room. Other considerations include flammability of the endotracheal anesthesia tube, the possible development of air pollution from particles of malignancies and infections, and the potential danger from impacts of pulsed lasers in miniseconds, nanoseconds, and even picoseconds.

We had particular concern with pulsed ruby lasers used in the treatment of metastatic melanoma. From tissue culture plates placed about the impact area, it was found that some of the plume fragments from lased animal and patient tumors were still viable. When controls of fluorochromes were painted on the skin of patients with tattoos, it was not possible to detect fluorescent particles in the environment after pulsed ruby laser impacts. With current laser surgery, continuous wave (CW) impacts are primarily used and are accompanied by minimal environmental pollution. However, pulsed laser impacts continue to be of interest in regard to the minimal production of radiation and transmission of heat in adjacent tissue.

Medical application

This new physical modality with selective absorption in the visible light range suggested the possibility of using lasers as a treatment modality. The initial experiments on living tissues were done with the laser microirradiation on tissue cultures, in animal eyes, on skin, and on tumors, especially melanomas. The initial clinical investigative experiments were done on pigmented spots, on melanomas, tattoos, café-au-lait spots, and angiomas.

There was an initial lack of interest in the development and support of laser surgery by the government, industry, and the armed forces. The seven-year support by the John A. Hartford Foundation of the Laser Medical Laboratory, Children's Hospital Medical Center, University of Cincinnati supplied the initiative for the research and development of medical applications of the laser. Surgeons became more interested where laser beams were continuous rather than pulsed. Now they felt they had, as it were, an optical scalpel.

The CO₂ laser

Photoexcision was possible first with the CO_2 laser and later with the Nd:YAG and then the argon laser. The original studies consisted of excisional surgery of animal melanomas. Low-output CO_2 lasers were used for the volatilization of inoperable metastatic melanomas, and later, higher-output CO_2 lasers were used for excisions. The various factors concerned in laser surgery included type of laser, power output, speed of excision, tension of the target, and its vascular supply. With the ruby laser, the argon, and to some extent the Nd:YAG, color properties of the target area also were important. However, because the CO_2 laser wavelengths are in the far-infrared, the color of the target area was not of any great significance for laser surgery, but the vascular supply was. With CO_2 lasers at the focal point, with small spot size and high output, precise excisional surgery was possible. With an out-of-focus beam and larger spot size, hemostasis was possible, especially for capillary oozing.

After animal tumor surgery we proceeded to liver surgery. Of interest here was an attempt to see what could be done for trauma to the liver, especially after the impact of the accidents resulting from automobile seat buckle. Excisional surgery of portions of the liver were carried out and, as stated, it was possible to control capillary oozing with the defocused CO_2 laser beam. Blood vessels larger than 2 mm diameter required clamping.

The next development of importance in laser surgery was the addition of the attached microscope. Attached to the CO_2 laser, this helped in the use of this laser for lesions of the oral pharynx and larynx and later for operative endoscopy. There then followed developments in gynecologic surgery including the treatment of intraepithelial neoplasia on the cervix and vagina and microscopic CO_2 surgery on the fallopian tubes for fertility. In out studies, the CO_2 laser was superior to the high-frequency electrosurgical unit for treatment of condylomata acuminata, especially for the giant condylomata (Buschke–Lowenstein) and condylomata acuminata in the pregnant woman. Increasing interest in fiberoptics has made it possible to transmit far-infrared laser beams, increasing the flexibility of CO_2 lasers for endoscopic surgery.

The argon laser

Early development of the argon laser showed its superior absorption by hemoglobin with consequent use of the previously untreatable and disfiguring port wine stain. The new microscope attachments now also made this a superior tool for fine vascular surgery, such as for telangiectasia of the face and for early rhinophyma [3,4].

Present status of medical lasers

Most of the effort in recent times has been in increasing the reliability and lowering the cost of the instruments used in laser surgery. The ruby laser continues to be used, especially in Japan, but not as frequently as the CO_2, Nd:YAG, and argon. Experiments with the CO and holmium laser have not been continued on any large scale. New developments in the CO_2 laser, the radio frequency (RF) and direct current (DC) waveguide types, and the Q-switched, are of considerable interest and importance. Also additional studies continue to be carried out, particularly in oncology, with the laser as an adjuvant for other techniques. Laser-induced fluorescence with hemato-porphyrin derivatives has been developed for diagnosis and treatment of early pulmonary cancer, and with increased absorption by tumors, it can also be used for the treatment of skin cancer. This technique has been used in China to attempt to differentiate between malignant and nonmalignant ulcerations. For laser surgery it has become possible in some fields, such as neurosurgery and gynecology, to define when this technique is obligatory, when it is preferable, and finally, when it should not be used. In the recently formed American Society of Laser Medicine and Surgery, there have been 12 separate surgical speciality divisions established, each headed by a laser surgeon with expertise in that speciality.

A field loosely called laser biomedical stimulation has developed in which there is world-wide interest. Low-output laser systems—helium–neon, helium-–cadmium, krypton, and probably copper vapor lasers—are used variously for presumed laser immunostimulation or as immunosuppressive agents in the treatment of arthritis, chronic ulcers, chronic infections, and even for acupuncture. Unfortunately, only with the arthritis program have adequate controls been done.

Other applications of lasers to medicine

Another field of laser medicine has also developed—the laser as a diagnostic tool and a precise laboratory analytical instrument. We did initial studies with laser transillumination to assess whether the passage of laser beams through tissue would be able to outline masses of different densities such as foreign bodies and tumors. Initial experiments were done with the helium–neon and krypton lasers and now we are using dye lasers and low-output Nd:YAG lasers. With the argon laser, image intensifiers, image transformations to visible images, and special photographic techniques are also used. However, the present imagery for laser transillumination is still inferior to that of mammography and xerography. Lasers are also under study to develop a type of CAT scan instrument.

The use of lasers for microemission spectroscopy followed next. This technique is being used extensively in industry, especially in ceramics and metalworking. Because of the lack of reliability, the dream of laser spectroscopy for quantitative analysis of cation determination from a single drop of dried blood on a piece of filter paper was not realized, although individual analyses of frozen skin biopsies for calcium, arsenic, and gold were accomplished. In Europe, this technique has been used in forensic medicine. Such methods have been used to study air pollution for carcinogens in occupational exposures and for the detection of narcotic drugs.

Laser cytofluoremetry utilizes the argon laser for scanning of stained single cells and has been developed into mass examination programs for Pap smear determinations. The same technique is used in cell-sorter systems now important in monoclonal antibody determinations in hybridoma technology. Other diagnostic fields include laser particle size measurement techniques, and the laser nephelometer [5] used for the determination of immunoglobulins such as rheumatoid factor. The studies of Kaiser [6] with the infrared lasers and special prisms have shown the practical value of lasers for measurement of blood electrolytes and other components. Laser Doppler velocimetry can now be used to measure blood flow by means of a simple probe that rests on the lip.

Laser dentistry in the United States has not developed as extensively as in Germany. We have done preliminary studies in laser dentistry for its effects on caries, tartar, and pulp cavities. There appears still to be great potential in the CO_2 vitrealization of dental enamel to prevent infection.

The newest field of laser medicine is concerned with the application of the revolution in laser communications and information handling to the treatment of patients and the teaching of medicine. There are extensive programs in industry and in the military but it has been very difficult to adapt these to medicine. Laser information handling and communication, made possible through fiberoptic communication systems, have great potential not only for in-house communication but also for the better delivery of health care to areas outside the hospital center. Laser discs may also have great application for the student of medicine. These past two decades of laser medicine and surgery have shown great progress and show great promise for the future.

References

1. Goldman, L., Rockwell, R. J., Jr. *Lasers in Medicine.* New York: Gordon and Breach, 1971.
2. Goldman, L., Richfield, D. The effects of repeated exposures to laser beams. *J. Invest. Dermatol.* 1965; **44**:69.

3. Goldman, L., Dreffer, R., Rockwell, R. J., Jr. *et al*. Treatment of port wine marks by argon laser. *J. Dermatol. Surg. Oncol.* 1976; **2**:385–8.
4. Apfelberg, D. P., Maser, R. M., Lash, H. Argon laser treatment of cutaneous vascular abnormalities: progress report. *Ann. Plast. Surg.* 1978; **1**:14–8.
5. Goldman, J. A. Investigative studies of laser technology in rheumatology and immunology. In: Goldman L, ed. *The Biomedical Laser. Technology and Clinical Applications*. New York: Springer-Verlag, 1981:293–311.
6. Kaiser, N. Personal communication.

SECTION II
Interaction of Lasers with the Skin

Cutaneous Laser Therapy: Principles and Methods
Edited by K. A. Arndt, J. M. Noe, and S. Rosen
© 1983 John Wiley & Sons Ltd

2

The Physics of Lasers

Donna B. C. Bourgelais and Irving Itzkan

This chapter is written to provide some understanding of the basic principles of laser physics. Lasers are rapidly finding acceptance as a tool by the medical community. Increased understanding of lasers by physicians, biomedical scientists, and other health-care personnel will undoubtedly result in new areas of application and modifications of existing procedures. Those readers interested in a more detailed presentation are referred to the overview by Leone and Moore [1] or the textbooks by Lengyel [2] and Siegman [3].

This chapter will compare and contrast lasers with more traditional light sources in terms of such characteristics as directionality, spectrum, brightness, and coherence. Certain parameters important for the full characterization of a laser will be defined and illustrated as will others required for an adequate description of laser application to tissue. Illustrations of the basic components

13

of lasers in common use will be presented, with emphasis on those already used in dermatology or, in the view of the authors, presenting great promise for future applications. Finally, a brief discussion of laser power-delivery systems and of practical considerations important for those planning to install a laser facility will be presented.

Comparison of lasers with traditional light sources

Traditional light sources such as a candle, or light bulb, radiate light in all directions. Some directionality may be provided by accessories, such as the parabolic reflector in a flashlight, or a Fresnel lens in a lighthouse or traffic light. By contrast, the light emerging from a laser is generally constrained to a narrow beam which propagates long distances with minimal spreading. This property, known as spatial coherence, is discussed in greater detail later.

Lasers provide a level of brightness far in excess of that available from traditional light sources. The accepted unit of measure for brightness is given in terms of power per unit area per unit solid angle, or watts (W) per square centimeter (cm^2) per steradian. In these units a typical incandescent bulb has a brightness of 0.1, the sun 1000, and an argon laser 1,000,000,000. This increase in brightness results, not from the change in total power made available from the source, but from the confinement of that power to a narrow beam. This property of the laser beam, which permits propagation over long distances with minimum spreading or focusing to a very small spot, is called spatial coherence. The small amount of spreading of the light beam that does occur is termed divergence; this will be discussed in greater detail in a later section.

Visible radiation is that portion of the electromagnetic spectrum to which the human eye is sensitive. It covers the wavelength range from 400 to 700 nm (nanometers). Longer wavelength radiation, from 700 nm to about 1 mm (millimeter), is referred to as infrared. Still longer wavelength radiation is classified as microwave. Radiation on the short side of visible, from 100 to 400 nm, is called ultraviolet. Beyond ultraviolet (wavelengths shorter than 100 nm) is the regime of X-rays. Conventional light sources emit radiation over a broad band of wavelengths, frequently spanning the entire visible spectrum. The spectrum, or range of wavelength, for incandescent light bulbs includes the visible and near-infrared, while fluorescent lamps radiate predominantly in the visible and near-ultraviolet. Lasers, on the other hand, usually have very narrow spectra. A range of wavelengths from a given laser may be as broad as 10–20 nm or as narrow as 10^{-3} nm. A light source whose spectrum covers the entire visible spectrum is seen as white while a narrow spectrum is perceived as a 'pure' color and referred to as monochromatic. For example, a typical helium–neon laser which has a spectrum peaked at 633 nm and only 10^{-3} nm wide appears red, while incandescent tungsten filaments and fluorescent lamps are seen as white or near-white. This laser property, narrow

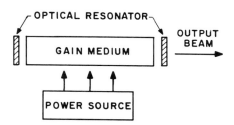

Figure 1   The basic elements common to all lasers are depicted here schematically. They may differ greatly from one laser to the next. The gain medium, for example, may be a solid as in Nd:YAG and ruby lasers, a liquid as in dye lasers, or a gas as in argon and CO_2 lasers

spectral emission, is often referred to as temporal coherence. It permits the radiant heating of selected chromophores, thus providing the possibility of high specific tissue damage.

Laser components

Figure 1 shows the basic components common to all lasers. The gain medium, which may be solid, liquid, or gas, accepts energy from the power source and stores it in the form of excited atomic or molecular energy states. A laser is usually designated by its gain medium. Photons travelling back and forth through the gain medium are reflected by mirrors which constitute the optical resonator. One of the two mirrors is partially transmitting, providing the laser output beam. As photons pass through the gain medium they interact with the atoms or molecules containing the stored energy and stimulate the emission of this energy in the form of more photons, hence the acronym *laser* (*light amplification by stimulated emission of radiation*). The emitted photons match the stimulating photons in wavelength, phase, and direction. This identity of properties, referred to as coherence, is the origin of the laser's monochromaticity and the ability to focus to very small spots.

The power source may be electrical, optical, or chemical. For electrical pumping, an electric field is imposed on a medium. This field accelerates charged particles (either ions or electrons) which collide with atoms or molecules, coupling some portion of their translational energy to vibrational or electronic states. CO_2, argon, and excimer lasers are examples of electrically pumped lasers.

One common form of optical pumping is a flashlamp. This usually consists of a quartz tube containing a rare gas (such as xenon) and two electrodes which allow a high-density electric discharge to pass through the gas. The resultant emitted light is then coupled into the laser gain medium using some form of reflector. Ruby, Nd:YAG, and flashlamp-pumped dye lasers utilize this form of optical pumping. Another form of optically pumped laser is the laser-pumped laser, in which a second laser serves as the optical pump for the laser gain medium. The argon laser-pumped dye laser is an example of this type of system. In chemically pumped lasers the energy stored in the gain medium is created by chemical reactions within it. An example of this type of laser is the HF laser where hydrogen and fluorine react to provide the vibrationally excited HF molecules.

Laser power delivery

Laser power is delivered through fiberoptic wands or articulated arms. In the wand, light travels through a highly transparent and fairly flexible fiber or fiber bundle. This system is usually lightweight and easily supported in the operator's hand. Fiberoptic delivery systems are used for lasers in the visible and near-infrared portions of the spectrum such as argon, dye, and Nd:YAG lasers. An articulated arm is a delicately engineered system of interlocking rotating joints, tracking mirrors, and protective cylinders which, though bulky in appearance, can often provide as much flexibility as the fiber wand. Since the system is counterbalanced, the operator does not support any of its weight. Articulated arms are used for lasers such as CO_2 in the far-infrared portion of the spectrum where fiberoptics that are presently available have poor transmission. Both wands and articulared arms are terminated in handpieces which incorporate focusing optics and sometimes alignment beams or additional safety shutters. Often the handpiece is removable and interchangeable with other units, providing varying laser spot size. A foot pedal may be provided as an additional control on laser power.

Laser characterization

Temporal behavior and emission spectrum

Lasers may be divided into two major classes by their temporal behavior. If the laser light is emitted continuously with little or no variation in output power it is called a CW (continuous wave) laser. Pulsed lasers are those whose radiation is emitted in bursts or pulses of light separated by intervals without light emission. Pulsed lasers may be further divided into single-pulse lasers which provide a single pulse of energy for each operator-controlled trigger, and repetitively pulsed lasers which provide a chain of pulses with a constant time interval between pulses. This is illustrated in Figure 2.

There are several important parameters required to describe the temporal behavior of a pulsed laser. These are shown in Figure 2. The repetition rate is the number of laser pulses emitted per second. For any given laser the repetition rate is limited by a minimum recovery time which is usually related to an inherent physical property of that laser. The temporal pulse width is often

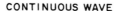

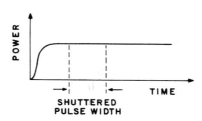

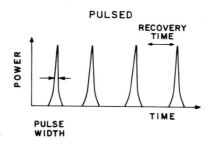

Figure 2   CW lasers provide continuous laser irradiation which may be gated on and
off with a mechanical or electronic shutter. Pulsed lasers provide short pulses of light
with a repetition rate that is ultimately limited by an inherent recovery time

given as the interval of time in seconds separating the moment at which the
laser reaches half of its peak value as the laser turns on, and the moment that
the laser turns off. The peak power is simply the maximum power that the laser
reaches at some instant during a pulse. In some lasers the peak power varies
from one pulse to the next. This is commonly referred to as pulse height jitter.
Other forms of jitter that are sometimes encountered include variation in the
time interval between successive pulses or the temporal width of successive
pulses. Such variations become important if extremely accurate dosage or
timing is required in a laser application. The energy per pulse is, as the name
implies, the amount of energy delivered during a single pulse and is commonly
measured in joules (J). It is approximately equal to the product of peak power
and pulse width. The average power is the product of energy per pulse and
repetition rate. Clearly the average power will be lower than the peak power
since each pulse or burst of energy is followed by a quiescent interval. This is in
contrast to a CW laser whose average power and peak power are the same.

Occasionally a CW laser may be provided with a mechanical or electro-optical shutter which periodically interrupts the laser beam. This effectively
provides a pulsed laser whose temporal characteristics are defined by the
operation of the shutter.

As mentioned earlier, the emission spectrum of a laser is generally confined to a narrow band of wavelengths although some lasers have multiple emission bands. An example of a laser that emits lights in a single, relatively broad band is the rhodamine 6G dye laser with an emission spectrum on the order of 10 nm wide centered at about 590 nm. When greater monochromaticity is desired, the spectral width may be reduced through the incorporation of additional optical elements. Other lasers such as the helium–neon mentioned earlier have inherently narrow spectral widths. The argon laser is an example of a laser with a spectrum consisting of multiple narrow emission lines. The major lines are centered at 488 and 515 nm and each is in the order of 10^{-3} nm wide. With suitable optical elements only one of the lines may be selected, providing a single-line argon laser. A Nd:YAG laser (neodymium: yttrium aluminum garnet) lases in the near-infrared in a single line at 1.06 μm (1060 nm) with a bandwidth of about 0.1 nm. CO_2 lasers are further into the infrared, at 10.6 μm (10,600 nm) and can have either a single line or a multiplicity of lines spanning 1.2 μm.

Divergence

Divergence is the angle that characterizes the spread of a laser beam as it propagates through space. In general, the divergence is composed of two parts, one of which can be corrected or eliminated with lenses. If the uncorrectable portion is reduced to the smallest value permitted by the wave nature of light, the laser beam is said to be diffraction limited. The smaller the uncorrectable divergence, the smaller the focal spot that can be achieved and, therefore, a diffraction-limited beam provides the highest attainable energy density. External optical delivery systems may also introduce significant amounts of divergence. For systems equipped with a fiberoptic or articulated arm delivery system, the terminator (sometimes referred to as the laser wand) produces a focal plane or minimum spot size at or near the terminator output aperture, and beyond this the spot size increases with distance. For a circulator laser beam, the cross-sectional area of the beam at any distance from the focal plane is given by:

$$\text{Area (cm}^2) = \tfrac{\pi}{4}\,[(d[\text{cm}] + 2\ell\,[\text{cm}]\tan\theta)]^2 \tag{1}$$

where d is the diameter of the circular spot at the plane of minimum spot size, ℓ is the distance from that plane to the skin or surface being irradiated, θ is the half angle beam divergence.

Both d and θ may be obtained from the laser system manufacturer or measured directly by the laser operator. Laser system divergence is usually quoted by manufacturers in milliradians (mrad) (1 mrad = 0.057°). The reader may recall that for very small angles, such as those encountered here, the tangent of the angle is approximately equal to the angle as measured in radians.

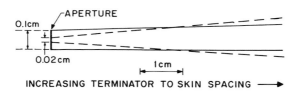

Figure 3 The solid line shows laser beam divergence for the 0.1-cm aperture, and the dashed line shows the greater divergence for the 0.02-cm aperture. At a distance of about 3.0 cm from the aperture, the beam diameters are approximately equal. For ease of illustration, the axis corresponding to distance has been compressed relative to the axis corresponding to beam diameter. (Reproduced with permission from Arndt, K. A., Noe, J. M., Northum, D. B. C., *et al.* Laser therapy. Basic concepts and nomenclature. *J. Am. Acad. Dermatol.* 1981; **5**:649–54. Copyright 1982, American Academy of Dermatology)

For example:

$$0.18° = 3.16 \, \text{mrad} \tag{2}$$
$$\tan (0.18°) = \tan (3.16 \, \text{mrad}) \tag{3}$$
$$= 3.16 \times 10^{-3}$$

Hence, the value of the half angle beam divergence, measured in radians, may be directly substituted for $\tan \theta$ in equation 1. This approximation is valid to within 5 percent for $\theta < 350$ mrad. To determine the beam divergence experimentally, measure the beam diameter at two different places along the path of the beam. The half angle beam divergence is then obtained from the formula:

$$\tan \theta = \frac{d_2 - d_1}{2\chi} \tag{4}$$

where d_2 is the diameter of the larger, more distant spot, d_1 is the diameter of the smaller, closer spot, χ is the distance between them.

For example, the Coherent System 1000 Dermatologic Laser is provided with two different terminators, both producing circular beams. The terminator with the larger aperture ($d = 0.1$ cm) provides a half angle beam divergence of 0.18°. For the terminator with the smaller aperture ($d = 0.02$ cm), the half angle beam divergence is 0.92°. This greater divergence implies that the beam from the smaller aperture spreads much more quickly than that from the larger aperture, as illustrated in Figure 3. The effect is so pronounced that for distances greater than about 3.0 cm from the terminator to the skin the laser spot size from the smaller aperture is actually larger than the laser spot size from the larger aperture.

Similar arguments apply for laser systems providing noncircular beam cross-sections (square, rectangular, etc.). It should be noted that if the output beam is rectangular, the beam divergence determining spot 'width' and that determining spot 'height' are not, in general, equal.

Irradiance, energy fluence, and exposure time

In order to develop an adequate understanding of the skin response to the laser radiation, it is necesary to note three characteristics of the laser application: irradiance, energy fluence, and exposure time. Irradiance [4] is simply the power density or power per unit area incident on the skin during a single pulse and is given by:

$$\text{irradiance} \left(\frac{W}{cm^2} \right) = \frac{\text{laser power output (W)}}{\text{laser beam cross-sectional area (cm}^2)} \qquad (5)$$

For example, a laser pulse with 2 W output and 0.1 cm diameter circular spot at the skin surface has an irradiance given by:

$$\text{irradiance} \left(\frac{W}{cm^2} \right) = \frac{2W}{\pi/4(0.1 \text{ cm})^2} \qquad (6)$$

$$= 255 \text{ W/cm}^2$$

The energy fluence [4] is the energy per unit area incident on the skin. For a single laser pulse of constant power, the energy fluence is the product of the irradiance and the pulse time as in:

$$\text{energy fluence} \left(\frac{J}{cm^2} \right) =$$

$$\frac{\text{laser power output (W)} \times \text{pulse time (sec)}}{\text{laser beam cross-sectional area (cm}^2)} \qquad (7)$$

Note that if irradiance and pulse time are specified, energy fluence is uniquely determined. For example, if the laser pulse time in the preceding instance is 0.2 sec, the energy fluence would be given by:

$$\text{energy fluence} \left(\frac{J}{cm^2} \right) = \frac{2W \times 0.2 \text{ sec}}{\pi/4 \times (0.1 \text{ cm})^2} \qquad (8)$$

$$= 51 \text{ J/cm}^2$$

As noted in the section on divergence, laser beams generally expand with increasing distance from the defined focal plane; thus, increasing the distance from the focal plane of the delivery system to the target skin increases the spot

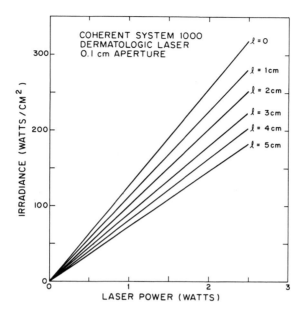

Figure 4   Shown above is irradiance as a function of laser power for several values of (ℓ) (terminator-to-skin spacing), a minimum spot size at the terminator of 0.1 cm, and laser half angle beam divergence of 0.18°. (Reproduced with permission from Arndt, K. A., Noe, J. M., Northum, D. B. C., *et al.* Laser therapy. Basic concepts and nomenclature. *J. Am. Acad. Dermatol.* 1981; **5**:649–54. Copyright 1982, American Academy of Dermatology)

size. This corresponds to decreasing irradiance. In Figure 4, the laser irradiance is plotted as a function of laser power for the Coherent System 1000 Dermatologic Laser with the 0.1-cm aperture and several skin-to-terminator distances. Similar data are given for the 0.02-cm aperture in Figure 5. Comparison of the two shows the effect of the stronger beam divergence in the case of the smaller aperture. For example, at ℓ = 5.0 cm using 1.0-W power, irradiance is approximately 70 W/cm² for the 0.02-cm aperture compared with about 150 W/cm² for the 0.1-cm aperture.

Spatial average energy fluence

Another important parameter in clinical practice is the total laser energy impinging on a given target area. Often the laser beam is swept across the target area with a speed selected by the operator to yield an apparently continuous skin whitening or tissue ablation.

For a pulsed laser without some uniform mechanical indexing, it is not obvious whether some laser pulses will overlap or whether there will be regions between adjacent pulses which are not irradiated but whiten due to heat

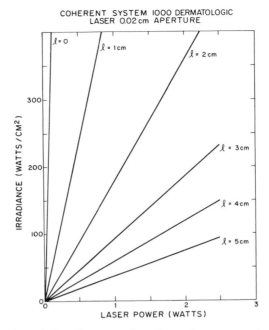

Figure 5   Shown above is irradiance as a function of laser power for several values of (ℓ) (terminator-to-skin spacing), a minimum spot size at the terminator of 0.02 cm, and laser half angle beam divergence of 0.92°. Comparison of Figures 3 and 4 shows the strong effect of the increased beam divergence associated with the smaller aperture. For example, with a terminator-to-skin spacing greater than about 3.0 cm, the irradiance for a given laser power is actually lower with the 0.02-cm aperture than with the 0.1-cm aperture. (From Arndt, K. A., Noe, J. M., Northum, D. B. C., *et al*. Laser therapy. Basic concepts and nomenclature. *J. Am. Acad. Dermatol.* 1981; 5:649–54. Copyright 1982, American Academy of Dermatology)

diffusion from adjacent irradiated regions. If the laser treatment has been uniform (with no areas skipped, gone over more slowly, or gone over more than once), this may be resolved by considering the total area irradiated and the total number of pulses delivered to that area. This yields the spatial average of the energy fluence over the treated area. Many pulsed dermatologic lasers are equipped with a pulse counter for measuring the number of pulses delivered. If no counter is available, the number of pulses is the product of laser repetition rate and treatment time. The area of the surface can be estimated before treatment by first outlining the region with a felt-tip pen and then tracing the area on paper that is sufficiently flexible to conform to the contours of the surface being treated. The area on the tracing paper may then be measured with a planimeter or by gravimetric techniques. Alternatively, a finely ruled graph paper, such as Keuffel and Esser 46 1513, may be used. Consider for example, a treated area of 3.1 cm^2 (a circle 2 cm in diameter) which is irradiated with a 2-W laser using 0.2-sec pulse time. The spatially averaged energy fluence is given by:

$$<\text{energy fluence}> = \frac{2W \times 0.2 \text{ sec} \times \text{no. of pulses}}{3.1 \text{ cm}^2} \tag{9}$$

where the symbol $<>$ is a common means of denoting an average value. If the spatially averaged energy fluence is given by equation 9 is greater than the single-pulse energy fluence given by equation 8, the operator has used overlapping pulses. In the other case (a spatially averaged energy fluence less than single-pulse energy fluence), there may be strong nonuniformities between the peak temperature at the center of each applied pulse and the peak temperature midway between irradiated spots. For many lesions, the threshold for scarring from laser therapy is so close to the threshold for permanent bleaching that these nonuniformities may result either in unbleached areas between the pulses (a mottled effect), or in excessive tissue damage and scarring from the high-peak energy fluence at the spot center. Both of these results are undesirable, and the operator should strive for a closer pulse spacing, reducing the laser power if necessary.

For a CW laser, the spatially averaged energy fluence is given by the product of laser power and exposure time divided by the total area irradiated:

$$<\text{energy fluence}> =$$

$$\frac{\text{laser power output (W)} \times \text{exposure time (sec)}}{\text{total area treated (cm}^2)} \tag{10}$$

For example, a CW laser operating at 25 W, swept continuously and uniformly over an area of 1 cm^2 for a period of 10 sec, would have an average energy fluence given by:

$$<\text{energy fluence}> = \frac{25W \times 10 \text{ sec}}{1 \text{ cm}^2} \tag{11}$$

$$= 250 \text{ J/cm}^2$$

It will be obvious to the reader that some of the parameters we have discussed are not independent. An adequate characterization of the laser therapy should, however, include at least the following information:

(1) irradiance (laser flux density) at the irradiated surface in W/cm^2;
(2) laser beam cross-sectional area and shape at the irradiated surface;
(3) laser pulse duration or exposure time in seconds;
(4) pulse repetition rate (pulsed lasers) in pulses per second;

(5) treatment time segments and intervals between treatment times;
(6) total treated skin area in cm^2;
(7) total number of applied laser pulses or exposures; and
(8) the type of laser used and its spectral distribution.

Practical considerations

In installing a laser facility in a laboratory or clinic, a number of practical issues must be addressed. The electrical power required is often in excess of that available from standard wall plugs; multiphase or 220-volt service may be required. Cooling water of up to several gallons per minute is often needed. Laser systems that require high purity or deionized water generally specify compatible filters.

Replacement parts, maintenance, and consumables will vary from laser to laser. Some lasers require a continuous gas supply (generally supplied in compressed gas cylinders) and an appropriately vented exhaust system. Other lasers will require periodic flashlamp replacement or dye replenishment. Other lasers, notably some of the CO_2 and argon models, are designed to provide several years of clinical use without maintenance or service.

Like many other powerful tools, lasers constitute a hazard if improperly or carelessly used. Perhaps the most obvious danger is that of eye damage either from a direct hit with the laser beam or from a stray reflection. To eliminate this possibility access to the room should be limited during the laser operation, windows and air gaps around doors should be appropriately shaded, and all personnel in the laser area should be equipped with goggles designed for the specific laser in use. Rings, watches, and other shiny objects should not be worn or allowed to interrupt the beam. A vivid example of the consequences of failing to observe appropriate eye safety measures has been noted [5] and is highly recommended reading for all who find their safety goggles annoying. BRH (Bureau of Radiological Health) regulations [6] stipulate additional warnings and interlocks required in a laser facility.

Since many lasers utilize high-voltage components, installation should be carried out with the same care that would be required for other high-voltage electrical equipment such as X-ray equipment. Adequate grounding must be provided and service should be attempted only by qualified personnel. Dye lasers may incorporate a flammable and/or toxic solvent and operators should familiarize themselves with recommended clean-up procedures for dealing with an accidental spill. Lasers that utilize compressed gas should be carefully and periodically checked for leaks in accordance with the manufcaturer's instructions.

Summary

The unique properties of laser light, including monochromaticity, coherence, and brightness, arise from the manner in which the light is created by photons stimulating the emission of other photons within a gain medium. These properties allow the delivery of intense light beams providing selective, localized energy deposition. Although only two lasers, argon and CO_2, are in common clinical use today, others, such as Nd:YAG and dye lasers, are being used in research and clinical investigations and may soon become available as common medical tools.

References

1. Leone, S. R., Moore, C. B. Laser sources. In: Moore, C. B., ed. *Chemical and Biochemical Applications of Lasers*. Vol. 1. New York: Academic Press, 1974:1–24.
2. Lengyel, B. A. *Introduction to Laser Physics*. New York: John Wiley & Sons, 1966.
3. Siegman, A. E. *An Introduction to Lasers and Masers*. New York: McGraw-Hill, 1971.
4. *International Systems of Units* (SI). National Bureau of Standards Special Publication. 1972; **330**:9.
5. Decker, C. D. Accident victim's view. *Laser Focus*. **6**: Aug 1977.
6. *Regulation for the Administration and Enforcement of the Radiation Control for Health and Safety Act of 1968*. HEW Publ (FDA) 79–8035.

3

The Spectrophotometer and Measurement of Skin Color

Stephen Tang and San Wan

The spectrum in the natural form emerges from the rainbow. Its wonder led to mysticism; its understanding, to physics ... Ptolemaeus (136 A.D.) correlated refraction with the rainbow, transforming a phenomenon of faith into a matter of reason.

[1]

Skin color and the spectrophotometer

The color of skin may be of diagnostic significance in some dermatologic disorders and therefore its precise analysis is of both clinical and scientific interest. The use of painted color standards for this purpose has the drawbacks

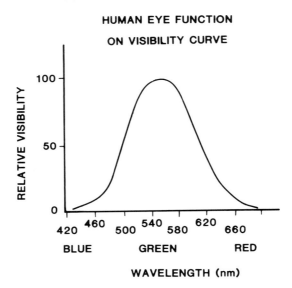

HUMAN EYE FUNCTION

ON VISIBILITY CURVE

Figure 1 'Visibility' curve from Coblentz and Emerson showing the sensitivity of the human eye for light of different colors. For normal eyes, green light (peak of curve at 555 nm) is the color most effective in stimulating vision. At the two extremes of the spectrum (blue and red), the sensitivity of the normal eye is poor. Coblentz, W. W., Emerson, W. B. *Bulletin of the Bureau of Standards*. U.S. Government Printing Office. 1918; **14**:167)

of observer variation (Figure 1). Spectrophotometry offers a more accurate method to specify color and to measure noninvasively the constituent pigmented structures of skin.

The development of spectrophotometry began in 1861 with Bunsen's ideas on spectral chemical analysis. Absorption spectroscopy has become popular since 1955 when Walsh demonstrated its advantages and devised simple apparatus for the analysis of biologic solutions. With this technique, characteristic light absorption peaks served as the spectrophotometric signature of specific chemical compounds.

One of the first dermatologic applications was a study by Edwards and Duntley [2] which involved the meticulous spectrophotometric study of *in vivo* human skin. The concepts explored included the dominant pigments of human skin, their anatomic and histologic distribution, and their variation by race. The authors concluded that:

(1) The major skin pigments of melanin, hemoglobin, and carotene had different and characteristic spectral curves.
(2) These pigments were largely segregated to various anatomic structures and could serve as chromophore markers for these structures.

DUAL BEAM SPECTROPHOTOMETER

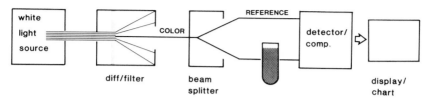

Figure 2 Schematic of the dual-beam absorption spectrophotometer used in usual laboratory analysis

(3) Therefore, examination of spectral curves could identify the underlying chromophores from the pigment admix and lead to an evaluation of their approximate quantity.

(4) Significant variation existed over different regions of an individual's anatomy and between individuals of different races.

This study was done before the mathematical tools existed to optically describe human skin and therefore did not allow quantitative evaluation of the chromophore and its associated anatomic correlate. General mathematical modeling of multilayer materials was developed by Kubelka [3] and was recently applied to model skin by Wan, Anderson, and Parrish [4] and Dawson *et al.* [5]. These studies are highly useful in providing both the theoretical considerations and the experimental demonstration of spectrophotometric analysis of *in vivo* skin. They also suggest specific applications to noninvasively quantify individual constituents such as the cutaneous blood concentration.

Current technology has contributed to the ease and speed of measurement utilizing fiberoptics, electronic sensors, and on-line computer processing—integrated with and expanding the potential applications of the traditional spectrophotometer.

The absorption spectrophotometer

This traditional instrument is composed of the functional components shown in Figure 2. The instrument shown is a dual-beam spectrophotometer. Single-beam units are available, but provide less resolution. A source of white light is filtered or diffracted into a component color (wavelength) and two equal beams are created. One beam (reference) travels unimpeded to a detector where it is compared with the other beam which has traversed a specimen solution. The relative change in intensity is expressed as percent absorption. Common ranges of wavelengths used in spectrophotometry span the ultraviolet to the infrared. Either a single wavelength is used and a single absorption or transmittance percentage displayed, or a range of wavelengths is used and a graph of wavelength versus absorption or transmittance percentage is plotted. This graph represents the spectral curve for the admix of chromophores of the solution with their characteristic absorption peaks.

Adaptation of the spectrophotometer for the study of *in vivo* skin

The major problem in the spectral measurement of *in vivo* skin is the lack of an appropriate intra- or subcutaneous detector for light that has traversed the skin. A secondary problem is the awkwardness of accessing parts of the human subject not near the viewing ports fixed to the spectrophotometer. These difficulties have been overcome through:

(1) measurement of reflected light from the subject with comparison with reflected light from a white standard.
(2) fiberoptic extensions from the viewing ports of the spectrophotometer to the actual measuring appliance.

Thus, the source light is delivered over fiberoptic conduits to the subject's skin. Two major schema have been used:

(1) delivery of specific wavelength(s) to the subject's skin with subsequent measurement of reflectance by photometer located either (a) at the skin appliance (Figure 3*a*, or (b) at the spectrophotometer, sensing reflected light returned from the skin appliance via fiberoptics (Figure 3*b*).
(2) delivery of white light to the subject's skin with subsequent sampling of reflected light by return fiberoptic conduit. This sample light is diffraction separated and measured for particular wavelengths (Figure 4).

Further variety of design is provided by the actual appliance with two major types that have been used:

(1) simple black chamber with an aperture for placement on the subject's skin (Figure 5*a*).
(2) white 'integrating' sphere with aperture for placement on the subject's skin (Figure 5*b*).

There are proponents of various configurations, but all share the common principle of measurement of light reflected from subject skin compared with light reflected from a white standard (100 percent).

Computerized processing of collected data offers ready interpretation of data and newer systems have built-in microprocessors to provide automated data collection, processing, and display. These systems are capable of using the modeling equations for the skin's optical structures and interpreting the

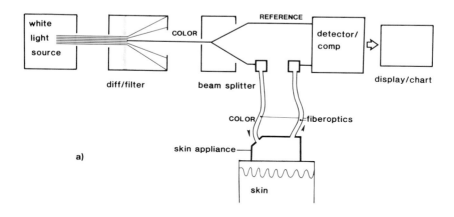

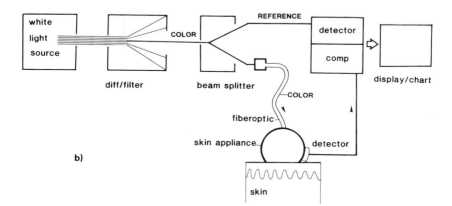

Figure 3   Schematic of spectrophotometer modified for reflectance measurements of skin. (*a*) shows the skin appliance connected via fiberoptic conduits to the spectrophotometer. (*b*) shows a similar arrangement except that the need for a return fiberoptic conduit is eliminated by use of a detector mounted at the skin appliance

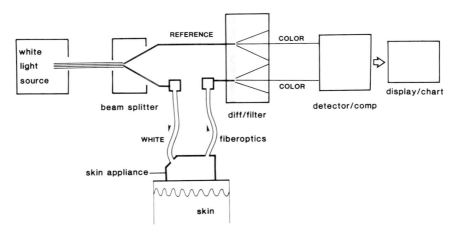

Figure 4   Schematic of spectrophotometer modified for reflectance measurements of skin. This arrangement differs from that of Figure 3 in that white rather than colored light is used to irradiate the skin. The reflected light is later diffracted and analyzed for its color components

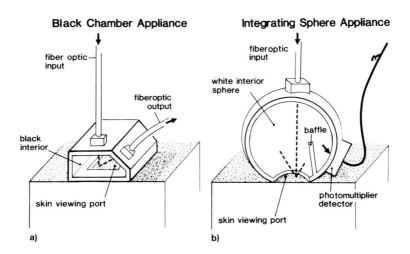

Figure 5   Two types of skin appliances: (a) has a black interior and measures a small fraction of the reflected light; (b) has a white interior and measures a much larger fraction of the reflected light from the skin

spectral curves in terms of absolute concentrations of pigments such as hemoglobin.

Basic optics of skin

Mathematical model for the optical properties of the skin

The normal skin is composed of the epidermis, and the dermis, the subcutaneous fat. The epidermis is approximately 100–150 μm thick and composed of closely packed epithelial cells forming microscopically distinct layers. It is the quantity of melanin in the epidermis that accounts for the racial difference in pigmentation. Beneath the epidermis the skin is supplied by a system of capillary loops that drain into two superficial venous plexi (SVP1 and SVP2) composed of blood vessels 40–60 μm in diameter. The capillaries are supplied by the superficial arteriolar plexus (SAP) formed by vessels 50 μm in diameter, which in turn originate from arteries entering the lower dermis. Both SVP and SAP run parallel to the skin surface. They form a horizontal mesh of vessels, the superficial plexus, which envelops the entire body surface and serves as one of the primary factors in general skin coloration. The lower dermis is composed of collagen bundles, elastic tissue, sweat glands, follicular structures, and blood vessels.

Optically, the skin can be considered to consist of three distinct layers:

(1) the epidermis,
(2) the upper dermis layer containing the superficial plexus, and
(3) the layer beneath the superficial plexus.

The major absorbing or scattering entity in each layer is melanin, blood, and collagen, respectively. This is a reasonable assumption, for though blood vessels are present in the lower dermis, the portion of visible light that is absorbed by hemoglobin (400–577 nm) does not penetrate below the superficial plexus. Consequently, the blood in deeper vessels contributes much less to skin reflectance than that in the superficial plexus.

In order to quantify major cutaneous chromophores (e.g. melanin and blood) noninvasively from *in vivo* spectrophotometric measurement (e.g. remittance), it is necessary to establish a relationship between *in vivo* spectrophotometric measurement and the optical properties of those skin component layers. The relationship turns out to be quite simple and is derived as follows.

First we must consider a sample made of two layers, shown in Figure 6. Light enters the sample and undergoes absorption and scattering within the two layers. The portions of light that leave the sample in the forward and backward directions are termed transmittance (T_{12}) and remittance (R_{12}) of the

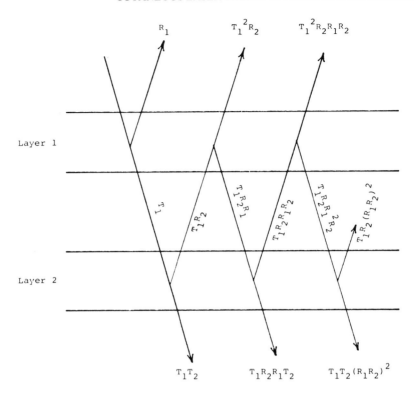

Figure 6 The two-layered optical model. R_1, R_2 and T_1, T_2 are remittance and transmittance of layer 1 and layer 2, respectively. The space between the layers is exaggerated to illustrate the interface. (Reproduced with permission from Wan, S., Anderson, R. R., Parrish, J. A. Analytical modeling for the optical properties of the skin with *in vitro* and *in vivo* applications. *Photochem. Photobiol.* 1981; **34**:493–9)

composite, respectively. They are expressed in terms of the remittances R_1 and R_2 and transmittances T_1 and T_2 of the component layers by:

$$R_{12} = R_1 \times \frac{T_1^2 R_2}{1 - R_1 R_2}$$

and

$$T_{12} = \frac{T_1 T_2}{1 - R_1 R_2}$$

respectively.

When the sample is made of three layers, the remittance (R_{123}) and transmittance (T_{123}) of the composite are represented by:

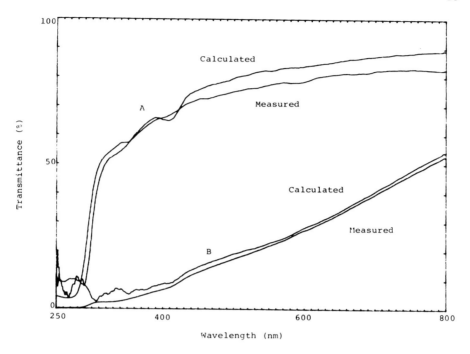

Figure 7 Comparison of measured epidermal transmittance with that calculated by the two-layer model. A = Caucasian; B = dark black. (Reproduced with permission from Wan, S., Anderson, R. R., Parrish, J. A. Analytical modeling for the optical properties of the skin with *in vitro* and *in vivo* applications. *Photochem. Photobiol.* 1981; **34**:493–9)

$$R_{123} = R_{12} + \frac{T_{12}^2 R_3}{1 - R_{12}R_3}$$

and

$$T_{123} = \frac{T_{12}T_3}{1 - R_{12}R_3}$$

Experimental verification of accuracy of models

The above quantitative model for the optical properties of the skin has been tested experimentally. Skin specimens were obtained from cadaveric abdomen and mastectomy material. The epidermis was separated from the underlying dermis after heating the skin in 60 °C water for 30 seconds. Transmittance of light through the epidermis was measured as well as calculated according to the quantitative model. Figure 7 demonstrates that the model is fairly accurate in predicting the transmittance of the epidermis. A more detailed discussion is given in reference 4.

Applications of optical models to quantify concentration of cutaneous blood

In addition to estimating the degree of epidermal pigmentation, the optical model has been used to quantify cutaneous blood [6]. By selecting three evenly spaced wavelengths, 544, 577, and 610 (the first two wavelengths correspond to the absorption maxima of oxyhemoglobin), the concentration of cutaneous blood in the superficial plexus expressed as ml/cm^2 can be approximated by:

$$\frac{1}{32.8} \left[\ln(R - r)(544) + \ln(R - r)(610) - \ln(R - r)(577) \right]$$

where ln = natural logarithm, R = *in vivo* skin reflectance, and r = minimum of R at 250–280 nm.

Derivation of the above formula utilizes the linearity of the logarithm of epidermal transmittance and dermal remittance between the wavelengths 450 nm and 700 nm. Consequently, the concentration of cutaneous blood so obtained is independent of the influence of epidermal melanin and dermal scattering. Using this technique, the measurements of cutaneous blood in the superficial plexi of the forearm and palms of 15 fair-skinned subjects were found to be 0.00736 ± 0.00159 ml/cm^2 and 0.01332 + 0.00384 ml/cm^2, respectively.

Clinical applications

Quantifying the pigmented components of skin can be useful in the assessment and treatment of selected dermatologic disorders. The examples that follow involve the assessment of hemoglobin content in the evaluation of port wine stain patients and in the treatment of patients with ultraviolet therapy.

Port wine stain (PWS) patients

Tang and Gilchrest [7] studied the curves of PWS patients, both lesional and contiguous skin as well as argon laser-treated lesional skin. In these patients the major lesional chromophore is the hemoglobin contained in the dilated superficial capillary plexus. Histologically, this plexus has been shown to dilate with age [8] and to respond to argon laser treatment by replacement with numerous undilated capillaries—a histological picture similar to the untreated lesional skin of juvenile PWs patients (see Chapter 14). Examination of the

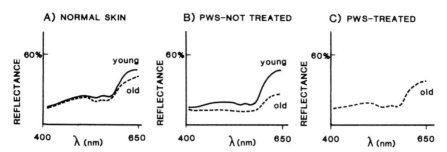

Figure 8   Spectral curves for normal, lesional, and argon laser-treated lesional skin of PWS patients. Normal skin of older subjects (> 40 years) shows increased absorption over young subjects (shift of reflectance downward). Untreated lesional skin shows an exaggeration of this shift. Treated lesional skin of older subjects closely resembles the spectral curve of untreated lesional skin of younger (< 20 years) subjects

spectral curves of 16 patients, aged 15–64, used a modified Carey 17 spectrophotometer and showed an age-related decrease in reflectance interpreted as primarily an age-related increase in the absorbing pigment hemoglobin (Figure 8a). The age-related changes in reflectance of untreated PWS skin showed an exaggeration of the shifts seen in normal skin (Figure 8b). These age-related changes cannot be explained by differences in oxyhemoglobin contamination only, but may reflect additional differences in other pigments such as reduced hemoglobin or in changes in cutaneous light-scattering constituents such as collagen. The spectral curves for argon laser-treated PWS were identical to those of untreated juvenile PWS skin for wavelengths between 400 and 600 nm, which is consistent with the histologic changes noted above (Figure 8c). These results and the work of Noe et al., where age, color, and percent filling of capillaries were closely correlated to therapy outcome (see Chapter 10) suggest a clinical role for spectroscopy in the assessment of PWS patients. It should be possible, using relatively simple equipment, to provide this capability in the clinical setting, offering a noninvasive and instantaneous tool to assess the treatment potential of the PWS lesion.

Erythema assessment in ultraviolet therapy

The treatment of various dermatologic disorders by ultraviolet light requires determination of dosage based on estimation of the subject's erythema dose–response curve. This estimation has traditionally relied on observation by the human eye which makes dose setting difficult and handicaps research efforts to develop more accurate dose–response curves.

Wan and coworkers [6] have demonstrated the feasibility of using the spectrometer to estimate erythema (cutaneous blood concentration) of the backs of six fair-skinned volunteers who were irradiated with doses of a broadband ultraviolet B source (Elder Pharmaceuticals, FS 36T12-UVB-

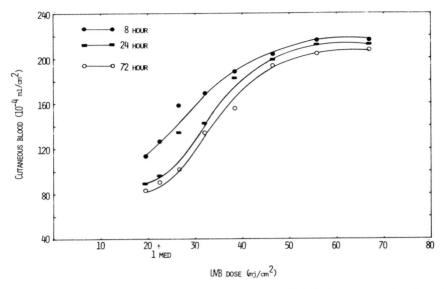

Figure 9   Quantity of cutaneous blood in the superficial plexus as a function of
            ultraviolet dose measured at 8, 24, and 72 hours after irradiation

HO-90°). *In vivo* skin reflectances at each site were recorded at intervals of 8, 24, and 72 hours after irradiation. The concentration of cutaneous blood in the superficial plexus was determined from the skin remittance by the formula given above. Figure 9 shows a representative dose–response relationship between uiltraviolet dose and cutaneous blood concentration. The relationship is 'S'-shaped and suggest a nonlinear erythema response most sensitive over a limited range of minimal erythema dose (MED). This specific range would vary between subjects and would be important to assess before setting a dosage level for treatment. Since Wan *et al.*'s method of estimating cutaneous blood requires only three reflectance measurements at the colors reflected for wavelengths 544, 577, and 610 nm, it should be possible to build a compact and inexpensive filter-based, electronically sensed, and microprocessor-operated 'erythema-meter' to be used in clinical practice. With such a device replacing erythema estimation by the human eye, it should result in more accurate and reproducible setting of dosage levels for ultraviolet radiation therapy.

Future applications

The method of quantifying cutaneous blood in the superficial plexus as described has many potential applications. It can be used to study redistribution of cutaneous blood during homeostatic control of body temperature, to evaluate the potency of topically or systematically administered vasoactive agents, to design new drug delivery systems in which synthesized liposomes filled with drugs undergo photolysis in the cutaneous vasculature of chosen skin sites, and to compare the erythemogenic effectiveness of various ultraviolet wavelengths.

The general quantitative optical model is also potentially capable of many other *in vivo* applications. The localization of most cutaneous pigments (melanin, bilirubin, beta-carotene, hemoglobin, and certain drug metabolites) in various layers of the human skin is known. Equipped with additional parameters of the pigments, e.g. the extinction coefficients, absorption maxima, and absorption minima (see Figure 2 in Chapter 4), we should be able to quantify the individual pigment *in vivo*, based solely on noninvasive optical measurements. Quantification of specific chromophores of laser therapy can also lead to better use of the ultimate specificity of the laser. Target structures of laser therapy can be analyzed by spectrophotometric means for absorption maxima relative to other structures not targeted for selection of the optimal laser wavelength(s) for treatment. This analysis could be done in the clinical setting with compact computer-driven devices. The technology exists today for all the applications discussed. Newer technologies in the future, such as Doppler ultrasonic probes or nuclear magnetic resonance, may be coordinated with spectrophotometry to yield an even more detailed noninvasive assessment of skin, its constituents, their individual functional states, and potential response to phototherapy.

References

1. Dawson, J. B. *Spectrochemical Analysis of Clinical Material.* Springfield, Ill: Charles C. Thomas, 1967: vi–vii.
2. Edwards, E. A., Duntley, S. Q. The pigments and color of living human skin. *Am. J. Anat.* 1939; **65**:1–33.
3. Kubelka, P. Optics of intensely light scattering materials. *J. Opt. Soc. Am.* 1948; **38**:448–57.
4. Wan, S., Anderson, R. R., Parrish, J. A. Analytical modeling for the optical properties of the skin with *in vitro* and *in vivo* applications. *Photochem Photobiol.* 1981; **34**:493–9.
5. Dawson, J. B., Barker, D. J., Ellis, D. J., *et al.* A theoretical and experimental study of light absorption by *in vivo* skin. *Phys. Med. Biol.* 1980; **25(4)**: 695–709.
6. Wan, S., Parrish, J., Jaenicke, K. Quantification of cutaneous blood by skin reflectance (abstr). *J. Invest. Dermatol.* 1982; **1978**:350.
7. Tang, S., Gilchrest, B. Spectrophotometric analysis of normal, lesional, and treated skin of patients with port wine stains (PWS) (abstr). *J. Invest. Dermatol.* 1982; **78**:340.
8. Barsky, S. H., Rosen, S., Geer, D. E., *et al.* The nature and evolution of portwine stains. *J. Invest. Dermatol.* 1980; **74**:154–7.

Cutaneous Laser Therapy: Principles and Methods
Edited by K. A. Arndt, J. M. Noe, and S. Rosen
© 1983 John Wiley & Sons Ltd

4

Considerations of Selectivity in Laser Therapy

John A. Parrish and R. Rox Anderson

The major therapeutic use of lasers in medicine is surgical. Even in the so-called nonsurgical specialities such as dermatology, the most frequent use of lasers is for removal or destruction of tissue. This is largely because the most striking feature of lasers is their high power; the high photon density effectively destroys tissue by thermal mechanisms secondary to the rapid rise in temperature in the absorbing tissue. Tissue can be removed by excision or vaporization or removed by host reparative processes responding to thermally induced necrosis. Although the exposed field diameter may vary from microns, e.g. on the retina, to centimeters, in all present forms of laser treatment the exposed tissue is rather uniformly treated and therefore affected as a contiguous target. Certain properties of the laser, however, create options for *selective* noncontiguous) effects on microscopic or even ultrastructural targets within exposed fields. Two mechanisms for achieving this type of selective effect include *in vivo* photochemistry and time-resolved spatial confinement of thermal effects.

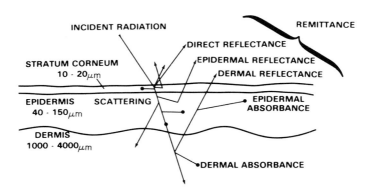

Figure 1   Schematic representation of optical radiation transfer in skin

Laser-induced thermal damage to pigmented biologic microscopic targets can be approximately modeled and the specificity, depth of treatment, and mode of damage can be predicted if the optical and thermal properties of the tissue are known. The specificity of damage to pigmented targets on a microscopic scale is controllable by appropriate choice of exposure parameters. The degree of confinement of damage to the target, the 'target' itself, and even the mechanisms of damage are in theory controllable by variation of wavelength and pulse width, and intensity. By consideration of these parameters, many of the problems associated with current laser treatments can most likely be diminished.

Skin optics

Knowledge of the optical properties of the tissue is essential to development of creative and specific laser therapy. Figure 1 is a diagram of the photon–tissue interaction options that occur when quanta impinge on the surface of the epidermis. Radiation may be reflected from the surface, scattered, absorbed within any layer, or transmitted to deeper layers. About 4–7 percent of ultraviolet and visible radiation is reflected at the air–tissue surface. Most of the visible radiation returning back from the skin has reached the dermis, from which it is back-scattered. Chromophores absorbing within the visible range include hemoglobin, oxyhemoglobin, and beta-carotene in the dermis and melanin in the epidermis (Figure 2). Note that melanin has increasing absorbance at shorter wavelengths. Absorption of radiation by the stratum corneum and by the whole epidermis is high for wavelengths shorter than 290 nm and is often maximum around 275 nm (Figure 3). This is because proteins, DNA, RNA, amino acids, and numerous other biomolecules absorb in this short-wave ultraviolet region. Scattering increases the average pathlength the photons must take to reach a given depth in tissue and increases their chances

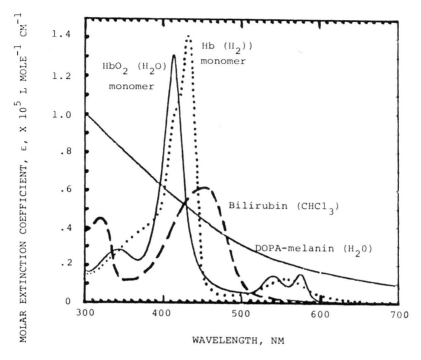

Figure 2 Absorption spectra of major visible-absorbing pigments of human skin. HbO$_2$ (——), Hb (...), bilirubin(-----), and DOPA-melanin(— · —). Parentheses indicate solvent. The spectrum shown for aqueous solution

of being absorbed before reaching deeper within the tissue. Scattering is also a function of wavelength; thus, shorter-wavelength radiation is scattered more. Hence, for ultraviolet and visible radiation, the longer the wavelength the deeper the transmission into skin. Table 1 describes radiation transfer to various depths in fair Caucasian skin as a function of wavelength [1].

The skin is perfused with arterialized blood well in excess of the metabolic needs of skin cells because the cutaneous vasculature is a heat-regulatory system for the whole organism. Therefore, an equivalent of the systemic blood volume may pass through the skin alone every few minutes. It should be kept in mind that ultraviolet radiation reaches the level of major cutaneous vascular plexi. Endothelial cells may be directly affected by the radiation, and blood cells passing through the skin may be photochemically altered.

Photobiologic principles

When a photon is absorbed, for some finite period of time the excess energy is invested in the absorbing atom or molecule, which is therefore said to be in an

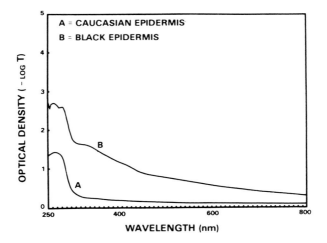

Figure 3   Absorption by Caucasian and black epidermis expressed as − log *T*, where *T* is the spectral transmittance as measured *in vitro*

Table 1   Approximate depth for penetration of optical radiation in fair Caucasian skin to various percentages of the incident density

Wavelength (nm)	Depth (µm)			
	50%	37%	10%	1%
250	1.4	2	4.6	9.2
280	1	1.5	3.5	7.0
300	4	6	14	28
350	40	60	140	280
400	60	90	200	400
450	100	150	345	690
500	160	230	530	1060
600	380	550	1270	2540
700	520	750	1730	3460
800	830	1200	2760	5520
1000	1100	1600	3680	7360
1200	1520	2200	5060	10120

Source: Modified from [1], with permission of the publishers.

'excited' state. The mode of this excitation depends upon the amount of energy invested (photon energy). At very high photon energies, such as x-rays, electrons may be removed from the absorbing molecule, resulting in ionization of the molecule. Infrared photons (longer λ, lower energy per photon) may alter lower-energy excitational levels by affecting rotational and vibrational states, resulting in changes most often recorded as heat. Absorption of visible and ultraviolet radiation may lead to electronic excitation—changes in the occupation of a molecule's electronic orbital shells, creating an excited 'electronic isomer' of the unexcited ground state molecule. All of these alterations must occur in discrete energy 'jumps'; hence the absorption of photons by molecules occurs at wavelengths with photon energies equal to those of the allowed rotational, vibrational, or electronic transitions of the molecules.

In skin or any other tissue, the biologic effects of absorption of optical radiation are caused by either or both of two basic mechanisms:

(1) responses to photochemical reactions; and
(2) responses to the heat caused by the nonradiative de-excitation and dissipation of the absorbed energy.

Most photochemical reactions have inherent specificity. Absorption is a precise phenomenon and the photoproducts produced from a given starting condition are often unique structures causing further specific reactions. The potential for specific dermatologic, hematologic, and immunologic therapies based upon *in vivo* photochemistry is both great and largely untapped. The activation of a specific, exogenously supplied, photochemically labile or reactive compound further expands capabilities. The example of hemato-porphyrin-derivative laser therapy of tumors (*vide infra*) is one example.

In contrast, the biologic effects of radiant heating are typically and comparatively nonspecific. Thermal damage to any one tissue or site follows one of only a few common mechanistic pathways regardless of the wavelengths used to cause the heating. The mechanisms by which heat damages tissues all derive from kinetic excitations, whereas photochemically induced damage derives from electronic excitations, often with little increase in temperature. Most cell types suffer reversible thermal damage over a relatively narrow range of tempertures near 40–45 °C, but can withstand somewhat higher temperatures for brief periods. Above approximately 50 °C, many proteins become unstable and tend to unfold, and membranes become more permeable. Between 80 and 85 °C most DNAs melt; this represents an effective upper limit for survival of active cells. Thermophilic bacteria can survive at 75 °C indefinitely, but mammalian cells are typically killed at temperatures around 45 °C or above. Vaporization damage occurs when water is boiled, near 100 °C. Thus, although photothermal effects in tissue are not strikingly specific, there is some range of damage mechanisms and sites.

To achieve a high degree of specificity for thermal damage to tissues, the specificity must be primarily spatial rather than mechanistic. Because of their high power, coherence, and monochromaticity, lasers are particularly suited for spatial confinement of optically induced thermal damage.

This chapter will focus only on new and experimental uses for lasers in dermatology and on considerations of information regarding mechanisms. The use of lasers in hematoporphyrin-derivative treatment of tumors will serve as an example of the creative use of the properties of the laser and knowledge of tissue optics to control *in vivo photochemistry*. Recent *in vivo* studies of the effects of tunable dye laser and XeF excimer laser on human skin provide a focus to discuss the possibility of selective *thermal* effects on specific structures within skin and potential advantages of not only the monochromaticity but also the narrow pulse width of some lasers.

Use of lasers in hematoporphyrin-derivative photosensitization treatment of cancer

The term 'photoradiation therapy' (PRT) is used by Dougherty and coworkers [2] to describe the use of a photodynamic hematoporphyrin derivative (HPD) and visible light to treat cancer. Since the first attempt by Tappenier and Jesionek [3] who used eosin and sunlight to cause regression of skin tumors, the concept of photoradiation therapy was not actively pursued until Diamond and coworkerse [4,5] showed that intravenous hematoporphyrin could be used to treat transplanted gliomas in rats. Acridine orange, a potent phototoxic dye, was also shown to cause tumor regression when mice were exposed to argon laser radiation after oral ingestion of the compound [6]. The first report of complete regression of experimental tumors due to selective phototoxicity in animals was with intravenous HPD and red light from a filtered xenon arc lamp [7]. Subsequent clinical work in humans by Dougherty *et al.* [8,9] has been aimed at finding optimal doses of HPD administered and defining the relative magnitude and duration of HPD-induced phototoxicity in normal and malignant tissues. Many case studies and small clinical series report the use of this therapy in a variety of tumor cell types.

The major shortcoming of current HPD photoradiation protocols appears to be tumor accessibility to the 630-nm radiation and it is probable that improved lasers and fibers will extend capabilities. Unlike previous arc lamp systems, the laser systems now being tested allow for photoradiation therapy of essentially any tumor accessible via endoscopes, intravenous catheters, or needles. Lasers provide means of delivering extremely high radiance monochromatic optical radiation through flexible optical fibers and therefore permit treatment through catheters, needles, or endoscopes. Further development of HPD or similar laser and photochemotherapeutic treatments depends in part upon advances in laser technology. The advent of tunable dye lasers and high-power ultraviolet and visible lasers open the most useful portion of the electromagnetic spectrum to a variety of innovative treatment possibilities. For example, in photoradiation therapy, laser systems operating near 635 nm, and focused into quartz fibers, are now being used to allow physical insertion of the optical fiber into a tumor mass. This results in more controlled and deeper delivery of the laser radiation specifically to the tumor mass.

The tissue necrosis produced by HPD photoradiation therapy appears to involve the production of singlet oxygen by one of several possible photochemical mechanisms [10,11]. HPD is widely distributed intracellularly prior to exposure [12] and singlet oxygen may act via a variety of radical intermediates to cause damage. Although other pathways leading to cell damage also occur, it is likely that oxidative alterations in the plasma membrane directly cause or promote cell lethality [2]. The properties of HPD which allow preferential retention in tumor tissue are unkown, as are the chemical identities of the photochemically active or fluorescent compounds of HPD. One major side effect of HPD photoradiation therapy is that normal skin remains photosensitive to visible light for weeks to months.

Selective thermal effects of lasers on pigmented structures in skin

Hemoglobin

Specific damage localized to skin microvasculature can be achieved using a pulsed organic dye laser operting at 577 nm [1,13]. Unlike other laser treatments, including those used in ophthalmologic surgery or coagulation where focusing of the laser is largely responsible for treatment specificity, tissue-specific damage can be achieved without focusing the laser upon a specific target. Rather, the optical and thermal transfer processes which ultimately govern the extent of the initial thermal damage can be modeled [1] and exposure conditions can be chosen for maximally selective heating of vessels during the laser pulse.

Wavelength of radiation should be chosen to maximize optical absorption by a target pigmented structure relative to other optically absorbing structures within the exposed tissue. Because radiation transfer depends on the optical properties of the tissue, the choice of wavelength will also determine the depth to which the optical radiation will penetrate with sufficient energy density to cause thermal effects.

For treating blood vessels, oxyhemoglobin is the logical target chromophore, because it is entirely intravascular and is the dominant hemoglobin species. If this chromophore is chosen, the wavelengths suitable for consideration are the HbO_2 absorption bands at 418, 542, and 577 nm. Despite the higher extinction coefficient of the 418-nm band, this wavelength is probably not as useful because at that wavelength penetration into the dermis is insufficient for exposure of vessels at depths greater than approximately one-tenth of a millimeter. Furthermore, absorption by epidermal melanin is higher at this shorter wavelength. If one uses the longer-wavelength HbO_2

absorption bands, less melanin absorption will occur. Therefore, a greater fraction of the incident energy will be transmitted to the dermis and less heating of the epidermis will result. The 577-nm waveband is an appropriate choice because extinction coefficients of HbO_2 at the 542- and 577-nm absorption bands are comparable, and the 577-nm radiation penetrates deeper into tissue than either 418- or 542-nm radiation.

Selective absorption of the 577-nm radiation by hemoglobin within vessels is excellent. Collagen, which composes 70 percent of the dermis by dry weight, and dermal ground substance have very low absorption of visible light [14] although the collagen fibers strongly scatter light. The wavelengths used with argon laser radiation (488, 514 nm) are located in a region between absorption bands of HbO_2, and within the absorption band for bilirubin, which is both itnravascular and extravascular.

Another consideration is the size of the target tissue. The size of the targeted structures should be commensurate with absorption of a significant fraction of radiation incident upon it. At 577 nm, the absorbed fraction of radiation incident on vessels of 50–100 μm can be estimated to be 80–95 percent, based on an effective hemoglobin concentration of 2×10^{-3} molar, and molar extinction coefficient of 6.08×10^4 at 577 nm [1]. For vessels of 20–50 μm diameter, the estimated absorbed fractions would be 45–80 percent, respectively. These larger vascular spaces are found in some patients with port wine stains.

The other critical variable in achieving selective microscopic thermal alternations is the pulse width—the duration of the exposure pulse. The laser pulse width modifies the extent of selective heating of tissue immediately surrounding the absorbing chromophores.

With relatively long exposure times such as those used in most dematologic argon laser treatments (> 50 msec), structures such as the epidermis that are some distance away from the target chromophore can be damaged due to thermal diffusion during the exposure. With long exposure durations, thermal damage will be extensive and nonspecific regardless of how carefully one has chosen a wavelength for heating of the target structure. This is because the thermal energy will have time to diffuse and be invested almost uniformly in heating of the surrounding tissue during exposure, despite its origin in the target structure.

On the other hand, if the incident energy is delivered within the time corresponding to retention of heat within the target structure, a maximum, transient temperture differential between the target structure and its surroundings will be achieved. After the exposure ceases, this localized heat in the target structure will then diffuse to surrounding structures, and in the process be dissipated over a greater volume such that the macroscopic temperature rise of the tissue will be much less than that achieved briefly in the target structure. The time associated with retention of heat within a target structure depends solely upon the size and thermal properties of the structure and its surrounding tissue. For blood vessels, removal of heat by blood flow must also be considered, but in most vessels this is a minor factor compared with radial heat flow for brief laser pulses [1].

Estimated thermal relaxation times for blood vessels of diameters from 10 to 150 μm cover the range of 0.1–10 msec, respectively. One would therefore expect a 577-nm laser with a pulse width less than approximately 1 msec to produce thermal damage confined to blood vessels. Other considerations of available energy at the level of dermal vessels, optical absorption, and heat capacities [1] predict that significant damage of vessels would require about 3–5 J/cm^2 incident exposure at 577 nm from such a laser.

As seen in Chapter 5, experimental results verify these theoretical considerations. Caucasian human skin was exposed to a dye laser operating at 577 nm with a 300-nsec pulse width and with exposure areas ranging from 2 to approximately 50 square millimeters [13]. The damage caused and the ensuing response are markedly distinct from the nonspecific thermal necrosis caused by argon, CO_2, or other reported laser exposures of skin by direct comparison [13]. Exposures of 2–4 J/cm^2 incident energy density from the dye laser immediately cause purpura, with no signs of gross damage to the epidermis.

Melanin

Similar reasoning and techniques can be used to select melanin as a target for specific spatially confined thermal alterations within tissue. Quantitative considerations of the optical properties of human skin, absorption spectra for natural melanins, and the size and thermal properties of pigmented cells within the basal layer of the human epidermis can be used to choose a laser with an approprite wavelength, pulse width, and energy density for producing selective damage to pigmented cells. This has been achieved in preliminary work by our group [15]. Guinea-pig and human skin *in vivo* and *in vitro* were exposed to single pulses from a XeF excimer laser (Tachisto) operating at 351 nm with 20 nsec pulse width. Grossly, the response consisted of an immediate wheal-and-flare reaction without purpura, followed by a sustained erythema confined to the site of exposure. After several days, mild desquamation with loss of pigmentation ensued.

Histologic observations (H & E and dopa stains) were made immediately and at 24 and 48 hours after exposure to a range of incident energy densities. These studies showed that cell necrosis was confined to the basal layer of pigmented Caucasian skin. The percentage of necrotic basal cells was dependent upon the incident energy density over the range of 100–400 mJ/cm^2 incident energy density. At 24 and 48 hours after exposure, signs of regeneration and sloughing were apparent. In albino guinea-pig skin, a larger incident energy density was necessary to produce histologic damage, but in this case the damage consisted of hemorrhage and necrosis localized to superficial dermal vessels, with little or no alteration of the overlying epidermis. The specific changes seen in human skin were not seen in the albino guinea-pigs because of the relative absence of melanin in the epidermis.

These studies strongly suggest that pigmented-cell-specific damage is possible using this excimer laser. Further work is in progress on the use of melanin as target. It is quite possible that organelles of the size of melanosomes could be specifically affected by selective laser therapy in appropriate wavelength and pulse duration. Other biochromophores and supplied exogenous biochromophores are also being studied.

Selective therapy with lasers

Capabilities for selective photochemical and thermal effects will increase as lasers, engineering, optics, and electro-optics become more sophisticated. But use of this equipment and expertise must be guided by experimental observations in normal and abnormal skin and by understanding of the mechanisms of laser therapy. Selectivity of effect on certain pigmented structures in skin may or may not be helpful depending on the pathophysiology of the abnormality being treated. Of greatest importance is the knowledge of the molecular and cellular mechanism of laser damage and subsequent host response which leads to therapeutic benefit.

For example, in treating port wine stains, if the goal of therapy is to induce total superficial tissue necrosis and subsequent host repair of the necrotic crater, then argon laser therapy of relatively long pulse duration may be most beneficial. If specific destruction of vessel integrity is most therapeutic then the tunable dye laser and pulse widths of less than 1 msec would appear promising. If maximum benefit is achieved by inducing perivascular fibrosis then slightly longer pulses might extend thermal alterations beyond the vessel to selectively affect and alter perivascular collagen. If uniform fibrosis is most advantageous then argon lasers or less specific targets may be considered.

In dermatologic uses of the laser, the same type of questions should be asked for treatments of tattoos. Is the goal to achieve tissue destruction of finely controlled depth under visual control? If so, then CO_2 lasers and relatively nonspecific water absorption could be most useful. If specific thermal or physicochemical alteration of pigment is the goal then other lasers might be chosen, considering wavelength and pulse duration. Laser-induced changes in the surface characteristics or particle size might change host response to the tattoo pigment. Thermal necrosis could be confined to a zone immediately adjacent to a tattoo particle. Other periparticle thermal alterations could be induced by selective heating of tattoo pigment and this could change the biologic material immediately adjacent to the tattoo pigment. Immobile but living pigment-laden macrophages could be killed. It may be advantageous to induce purpura or semiselective focal necrosis and expect the pigment to be removed by the host response. The degree of selective, intense, transient heating by pulsed lasers of certain targets is not in theory bound by temperatures or damage mechanisms tolerated by tissue. It may be possible or even likely that the extreme temperatures (hundreds of degrees centigrade) needed to oxidize or fragment tattoo pigments can be achieved, still without widespread destruction of surrounding biologic tissue.

Selective uses of lasers in dermatology, medicine, and surgery will increase but must be guided by good hypotheses, careful experiments, and good histopathologic studies defining goals and mechanisms of laser therapy of skin.

References

1. Anderson, R. R., Parrish, J. A. Microvasculature can be selectively damaging using dye lasers: a basic theory and experimental evidence in human skin. *Lasers in Surgery and Medicine.* 1981; **1**:263–76.
2. Dougherty, T. J., Weishaupt, K. R., Boyle, D. G., Photoradiation therapy of malignant tumors. In: de Vita, U., Hellman, S., Rosenberg, S., eds. *Principles and Practice of Oncology.* Philadelphia: J. B. Lippincott, 1982, in press.
3. Tappenier, J., Jesionek, A. Therapeutische Versuche mit fluoreszierenden Stoffe. *Munch Med Wochenschr.* 1903; **1**:2042–4.
4. Diamond, I., Granelli, S., McDonagh, A. F., *et al.* Photodynamic therapy of malignant tumors. *Lancet.* 1972; **2**:1175–7.
5. Granelli, S., Diamond, I., McDonagh, A. F., *et al.* Photochemotherapy of glioma cells by visible light and hematoporphyrin. *Cancer Res.* 1975; **35**:2567–70.
6. Tomson, S. H., Emmett, E. A., Fox, S. H. Photodestruction of mouse epithelial tumors after acridine orange and argon laser. *Cancer Res.* 1974; **34**:3124–7.
7. Dougherty, T. J., Grindey, G. B., Fiel, R., *et al.* Photoradiation therapy II. Cure of animal tumors with hematoporphyrin and light. *J. Natl Cancer Inst.* 1975; **55**:115–9.
8. Dougherty, T. J., Kaufman, J. E., Goldfarb, A., *et al.* Photoradiation therapy for the treatment of malignant tumors. *Cance Res.* 1978; **38**:2628–35.
9. Dougherty, T. J., Lawrence, G., Kaufman, J. E., *et al.* Photoradiation in the treatment of recurrent breast carcinoma. *J. Natl Cancer Inst.* 1979; **62**:231–7.
10. Weishaupt, K. R., Gomer, C. J., Dougherty, T. J. Identification of singlet oxygen as the cytotoxic agent in photo-inactivation of a murine tumor. *Cancer Res.* 1976; **36**:2326–9.
11. Moan, J., Pettersen, E. O., Christensen, T. The mechanism of photodynamic inactivation of human cells in-vitro in the presence of hematoporphyrin. *Br. J. Cancer.* 1979; **39**:398–401.
12. Gomer, C. J. Evaluation of in-vivo tissue localization in-vitro photosensitization reactions of hematoporphyrin derivative. Ph.D. Thesis submitted to the Graduate School, State University of New York at Buffalo, 1978.
13. Greenwald, J., Rosen, S., Anderson, R. R., *et al.* Comparative histological studies of the tunable dye (at 577 nm) laser and argon laser: the specific vascular effects of the dye laser. *J. Invest. Dermatol.* 1981; **77**:305–10.

14. Anderson, R. R., Hu, J. H., Parrish, J. A. Optical radiation transfer in the human skin and application in *in vivo* remittance spectroscopy. In: *Proceedings of the Symposium on Bioengineering and the Skin, Cardiff, Wales, July 19–21.* London: International Medical Publishers, 1982, in press.
15. Anderson, R. R., Parrish, J. A. Cutaneous effects of 351 nm excimer laser irradiation. Presented at the Second Annual Meeting of the American Society for Laser Medicine and Surgery, Hilton Head Island, SC, January 25–27, 1982.

Cutaneous Laser Therapy: Principles and Methods
Edited by K. A. Arndt, J. M. Noe, and S. Rosen
© 1983 John Wiley & Sons Ltd

5

Vascular Supply of Normal Skin and the Comparative Histologic Effects of the Tunable Dye (at 577 nm) Laser and Argon Laser on Normal Skin

Seymour Rosen

Lasers have been in clinical use in dermatology for ever 15 years for the treatment of a variety of cutaneous lesions. One of the initial studies reports the efficacy of the argon and ruby lasers in the therapy of port wine stains (PWS) [1]. Immediate histologic changes included diffuse coagulative necrosis of the epidermis and papillary dermis. Within 3 months after treatment, the skin became less violaceous, approximating normal skin color. Other physicians have documented the value of argon laser therapy of PWS in larger numbers of patients [2–5]. Argon laser therapy seems most effective in older patients with purple lesions containing ectatic blood-filled vessels [6]. In younger patients with pink lesions and small, relatively bloodless vessels, poor results and scarring are unfortunately common [6].

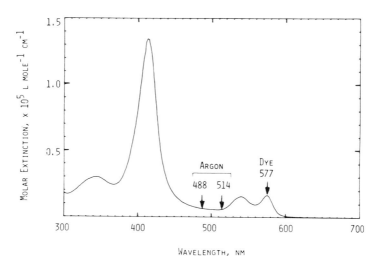

Figure 1   Absorption spectrum of oxyhemoglobin. Note that the argon emission (488, 514 nm) is at wavelengths not well absorbed by hemoglobin. The tunable dye laser was set at 577 nm to maximize absorption. The maximum absorption of hemoglobin is near 400 nm but this radiation is not transmitted as deeply into the dermis as 577-nm radiation. (From Greenwald, J., Rosen, S., Anderson, R., *et al*. Comparative histological studies of the tunable dye (at 577 nm) laser and argon laser: the specific vascular effects of the dye laser. *J. Invest. Dermatol.* 1981; **77**:305–10. Copyright 1982, The Williams & Wilkins Co.)

Lasers are capable of very high-power density, extremely short pulses, and virtually absolute monochromaticity. Because of their high-power density, absorption of laser radiation can lead to extremely high focal temperatures and result in coagulation necrosis or boiling of tissue. After therapy of PWS with argon, ruby, or carbon dioxide (CO_2) lasers, diffuse coagulation necrosis occurs throughout the immediately exposed field. It is possible, however, to utilize other properties of the laser to achieve photon–tissue interactions that are quantitatively and qualitatively different from those seen after exposure to conventional sources [7], and which also permit selective destruction of specific structures within skin [8]. Based on the optical properties of human skin and blood [8], the absorption coefficient of hemoglobin (Figure 1), vessel size, and thermal diffusion theory, the radiation at 577 nm should destroy blood vessels while sparing other dermal structures and the overlying epidermis [7–9]. This can be provided by the tunable dye laser, an instrument which allows high-power density, short pulse duration, and wavelength selection, and with rhodamine 575 dye is operated at 577 nm.

Vascular supply of normal skin

The vascular supply of human arm skin is diagrammatically depicted in Figure

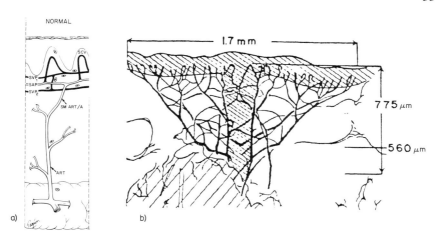

Figure 2 Schematic diagram of the microvasculature in normal human arm skin (*left*) and face (*right*). SCV = superficial capillary venule; SVP_1 and SVP_2 = superficial and deep layers of superficial venular plexus; SAP = superficial arteriolar plexus; SM ART/A = small artery/arteriole; ART = artery. (*Left*, from Dvorak, A., Mihm, M. C., Jr, Dvorak, H. Morphology of delayed-type hypersensitivity reactions in man. II. Ultrastructural alterations affecting the microvasculature and tissue mast cells. *Lab. Invest.* 1976; **34**:179–91. Copyright 1977, U.S.–Canadian Division of the International Academy of Pathology. *Right*, from Moretti, G., Ellis, R., Mescon, H. Vascular patterns in the skin of the face. *J. Invest. Dermatol.* 1959; **33**:103–12. Copyright 1960, The Williams & Wilkins Co.)

2*a* [10]. Medium-sized arteries present in the subcutaneous tissue branch just beneath the reticular dermis and from the *deep vascular plexus*. These then give rise to vertical branches whose caliber diminishes as they extend upward into the dermis. In the upper reticular dermis these vessels give rise to a plexus of horizontally oriented arterioles, the *superficial arteriolar plexus*. From this plexus, afferent branches arise, extend into the dermal papillae, loop and return to the upper reticular dermis, forming a superficial venous plexus that extends above and beneath the arteriolar plexus. Thereafter the venous circulation parallels that of the arterial.

The cutaneous vascular anatomy varies with region, but a detailed study of the vascular pattern of facial skin is available [11] (Figure 2*b*). This report found relatively consistent form and depth of the deep vascular plexus, which was located between 1.3 and 1.6 mm in the dermis. Regularly spaced branches from the latter plexus bifurcate between 560 and 775 μm and then continue to branch at 470, 360, 270, 180, 90, and 45 μm. The character of the branching is different with various facial regions (acute versus right angle). In essence, therefore, the facial superficial vascular plexus is almost completely contained in the upper 0.5 mm of dermis.

Experimental design and results

In order to compare the effects of argon and dye lasers on normal skin, a series of experiments was undertaken. Different sites of normal volar forearm skin of 10 healthy young Caucasian subjects were exposed to 10 pulses each of 300 nsec from a dye laser set at 577 nm [9]. The laser used was a coaxial flashlamp tunable dye laser with output capability of up to 0.5 J in a pulse width of 350 nsec (full width half maximum). The laser, supplied by Phase-R Corporation, was focused into a fiberoptic light pipe to produce spot diameters from 1 mm to 4 mm. The dye used was Yellow II (rhodamine 575) which was prism tuned to 577 nm. Energy density could be varied from 0.5 J/cm^2 by altering the voltage on the laser. Exposure field was 1 mm in diameter and exposure doses were varied by changing the laser power so that each subject had at least two exposures to 1, 2, 3, and 5 J/cm^2.

Single sites of normal volar forearm were subjected to 10 1-mm diameter pulses from an argon laser (Coherent Radiation Model No. 1000) in seven healthy young Caucasians in doses ranging from 12.5 to 40 J/cm^2. The argon laser emits radiation at 488 and 514 nm.

Gross clinical observations were recorded immediately, at 24 hours and at 48 hours. No anesthesia was used prior to the laser exposures. Trephine punch biopsies of exposed sites were performed: immediately in 12 instances, twice at 24 hours, and 16 at 48 hours (dye laser); immediately in seven instances and five at 48 hours (argon laser). Two percent Xylocaine without epinephrine was used for anesthesia. Biopsy specimens were fixed in formalin, dehydrated, embedded in paraffin, and cut at 4 μm thickness; hematoxylin and eosin, Masson trichrome, and elastic van Gieson stains were done. Two subjects were also tested with the dye laser tune to 590 nm; biopsies were not obtained at this wavelength.

Argon laser

Energies at less than 15 J/cm^2 (per pulse) produced no gross alterations, but at 20 J/cm^2 the skin imediately turned a whitish color. At 25 J/cm^2 and 30 J/cm^2, a white color followed by crusting 24 hours later was noted.

Histologically (Figures 3 and 4), immediate changes at lower dose levels were those of keratinocyte vacuolization. With higher doses, epidermal cauterization was present, adjacent to which a zone of keratinocyte vacuolization change was noted. Dermal collagen necrosis (cauterization) was regularly observed as distortion and basophilia in hematoxylin and eosin stains, iron hematoxylin affinity in elastic van Gieson preparations, and loss of ability to polarize. The depth of histologically identifiable necrosis varied from 0.125 to 0.3 mm of dermis; all cellular elements were destroyed within this zone with no preservation of structure. At 48 hours, the epidermis was necrotic and

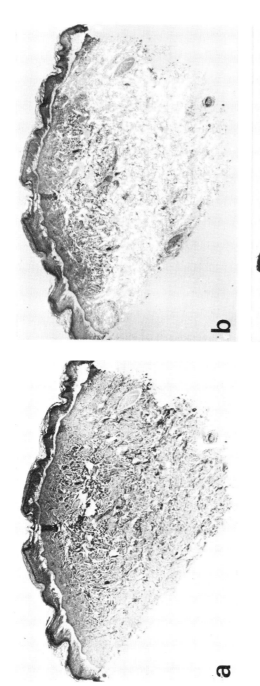

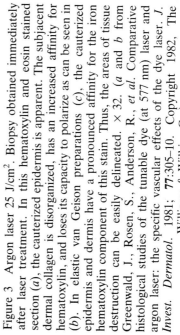

Figure 3 Argon laser 25 J/cm². Biopsy obtained immediately after laser treatment. In this hematoxylin and eosin stained section (*a*), the cauterized epidermis is apparent. The subjacent dermal collagen is disorganized, has an increased affinity for hematoxylin, and loses its capacity to polarize as can be seen in (*b*). In elastic van Geison preparations (*c*), the cauterized epidermis and dermis have a pronounced affinity for the iron hematoxylin component of this stain. Thus, the areas of tissue destruction can be easily delineated. × 32. (*a* and *b* from Greenwald, J., Rosen, S., Anderson, R., *et al.* Comparative histological studies of the tunable dye (at 577 nm) laser and argon laser: the specific vascular effects of the dye laser. *J. Invest. Dermatol.* 1981; 77:305–10. Copyright 1982, The Williams & Wilkins Co.)

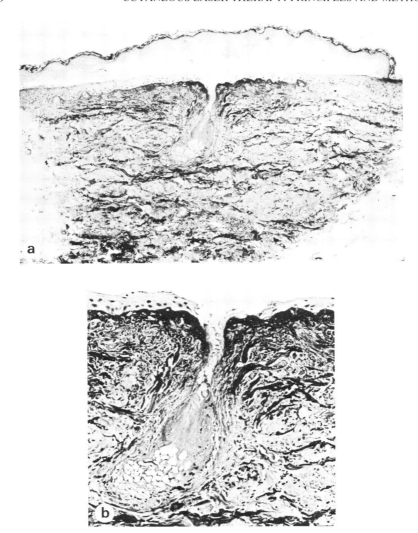

Figure 4   Argon laser 30 J/cm². In this biopsy obtained after 48 hours, the necrotic epidermis is readily apparent. Approximately 1 mm of epidermal regeneration has already occurred. The extent of collagen necrosis is easily discerned in the elastic van Geison stained sections (*a, b*) where it seems to invaginate and surround the upper aspect of the necrotic pilosebaceous apparatus. Although there is no adjacent collagen necrosis, the lower portion of the sebaceous gland is completely necrotic. *a*, × 40; *b*, × 91. (From Greenwald, J., Rosen, S., Anderson, R., *et al.* Comparative histological studies of the tunable dye (at 577 nm) laser and argon laser: the specific vascular effects of the dye laser. *J. Invest. Dermatol.* 1981; **77**:305–10. Copyright 1982, The Williams & Wilkins Co.)

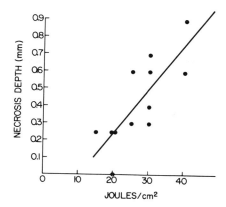

Figure 5   Relationship of depth of skin necrosis (epidermis and dermis) to energy applied with the argon laser. There is a good correlation between the amount of energy (J/cm^2) and depth of necrosis (Pearson correlation coefficient 0.82). (From Greenwald, J., Rosen, S., Anderson, R., *et al.* Comparative histological studies of the tunable dye (at 577 nm) laser and argon laser: the specific vascular effects of the dye laser. *J. Invest. Dermatol.* 1981; **77**:305–10. Copyright 1982, The Williams & Wilkins Co.)

completely detached; 1.0 mm of epidermal regeneration was observed. The collagen necrosis varied from 0.2 to 0.8 mm dermal thickness. The pilosebaceous apparatus was extensively necrotic both within and beneath the region of collagen necrosis. In the zone subjacent to the collagen necrosis, necrotic vessels and sweat glands now were also observed; a slight neutrophilic infiltrate was present.

Thus the initial response to present-day argon laser treatment is necrosis of epidermis and superficial dermis (see Figure 7). After 48 hours, cell death becomes evident in structures (vessels, sweat glands, and pilosebaceous apparatus) of the deeper dermal zone. The correlation between depth of epidermal and collagen necrosis and exposure dose is excellent (Figure 5). Only a mild acute inflammatory response was observed at the 48-hour period and no anatomic components were selectively destroyed.

Dye laser

In contrast to the argon laser, gross effects on normal skin were seen at much lower doses. At 3–5 J/cm^2, purpuric macules and papules were noted without apparent epidermal alteration. When wavelength was shifted from 577 to 590 nm, no changes in the skin could be observed at energies varying from 1 to 5 J/cm^2. Histologically, the primary alterations were largely vascular in nature and basically involved the superficial vascular plexus, sparing the ascending arterial and venular arcade. Clusters of tightly aggregated erythrocytes which had an orange hue were observed within vessels. Endothelial and transmural necrosis associated with rupture and hemorrhage was present (Figure 6). In a few biopsies, neutrophils were observed marginating and emigrating through the arteriolar and venous walls; no karyorrhexis was present. Such vessels had little endothelial alteration or vessel necrosis.

At 48 hours, the vessel walls were necrotic, replaced by fibrin; polymorpho-nuclear leukocytes and karyorrhexis were very evident, a pattern of 'acute vasculitis' (Figure 6). However, some superficial vessels demonstrated apparent reconstitution of endothelial cells. Hemorrhage was less striking than in the initial biopsies. The 'vasculitic' change occurred in the approximately upper 0.5 mm of dermis. In the deeper dermis (0.5–1.1 mm) a more diffuse, predominately perivascular polymorphonuclear leukocytic infiltrate was noted occasionally associated with lymphocytes.

The threshold energy for induction of significant vascular damage histologi-cally varied primarily from 2 to 3 J/cm^2. However, even at 1 J/cm^2 slight alterations consisting of minimal hemorrhage and erythrocyte agglutination were noted. Edema, hemorrhage, and slight neutrophilic infiltrate were the only dermal changes noted at these energy levels.

The threshold for significant epidermal alterations appears to be approxi-mately 3 J/cm^2, since energy levels of 1–2 J/cm^2 caused no epidermal changes. In biopsies in which 3 J/cm^2 had been administered, only small foci of epithelial cell necrosis were noted but, at 5 J/cm^2, full-thickness epidermal necrosis and subepithelial blister formation were apparent. At this energy level, the most severe vascular damage was present. However, necrosis of collagen, pilosebaceous apparatus, and sweat glands was never seen.

Thus, the initial response to dye laser treatment is an erythrocyte aggregation, vessel rupture, and hemorrhage (Figure 7). At 48 hours, a pattern similar to that observed in acute vasculitis is present in the upper dermis (0.5 mm thickness), but a primarily perivascular neutrophilic infiltration is observed fully 1.0 mm beneath the epidermis. Epidermal necrosis was present only in some of the biopsies, despite conspicuous vascular damage. Necrosis of the pilosebaceous apparatus, sweat glands, and collagen was not observed.

Discussion

By using laser radiation of appropriate wavelength, pulse duration, and peak power, dermal blood vessels can be selectively damaged. This effect appears to depend on both the wavelength and pulse duration of the dye laser. A setting of 577 nm was chosen so that hemoglobin in vessels would absorb the radiation. Although hemoglobin absorbs maximally near 420 nm this radiation is not transmitted as deeply into dermis as radiation at 577 nm, a lesser hemoglobin absorption band. When the dye laser was tuned to 590 nm, no vessel damage was seen at energy levels that severely affected vessels at 577 nm. The pulse

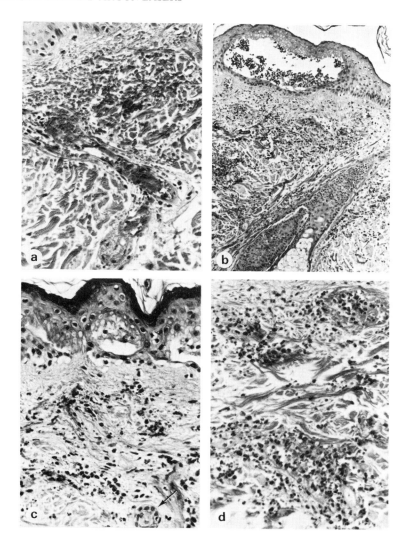

Figure 6 The immediate effect (*a*) of the dye laser is erythrocyte aggregation, vessel rupture, and hemorrhage. After 48 hours, epidermal changes, vesicle formation, and necrosis were seen in some biopsies (*b, c*). The most obvious changes were those of a pattern similar to an acute necrotizing vasculitis (*b, c, d*). Note the preservation of the pilosebaceous apparatus and the eccrine duct (*arrow*), in spite of the adjacent severe vascular damage. Dye laser at 577 nm, 3–5 J/cm². Hematoxylin and eosin. *a*, × 190; *b*, × 80; *c*, ×176; *d*, ×247. (*a–c* from Greenwald, J., Rosen, S., Anderson, R., *et al.* Comparative histological studies of the tunable dye (at 577 nm) laser and argon laser: the specific vascular effects of the dye laser. *J. Invest. Dermatol.* 1981; **77**:305–10. Copyright 1982, The Williams & Wilkins Co.)

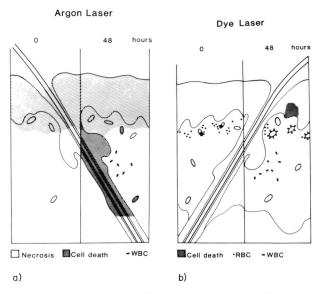

Figure 7   Diagrammatic comparison of the relative effects of the argon and dye laser. The initial response of the argon laser (*a*) is diffuse epidermal and dermal necrosis. After 48 hours, deeper thermal injury is reflected by cell death and a mild polymorphonuclear response. In sharp contrast, the initial response to the dye laser (*b*) is erythrocyte aggregation, vessel rupture, and hemorrhage. After 48 hours, a vasculitic pattern is present in the upper epidermis. Focal epidermis necrosis is variably seen. The energy required to elicit these changes by the dye laser is 3 J/cm^2 in contrast to the argon laser where at least 15 J/cm^2 is required. (From Greenwald, J., Rosen, S., Anderson, R., *et al*. Comparative histological studies of the tunable dye (at 577 nm) laser and argon laser: the specific vascular effects of the dye laser. *J. Invest. Dermatol*. 1981; **77**:305–10. Copyright 1982, The Williams & Wilkins Co.)

width of the dye laser is 350 nsec, a short time compared to the calculated thermal relaxation ('cooling') time of 1 msec for structures the size of ectatic PWS vessels. Although heat-induced changes would be expected to be largely confined to the absorbing chromophore, there was evidently sufficient energy transfer to damage and destroy vascular walls. In sharp contrast, the present-generation argon laser is not at a wavelength absorbed as well by hemoglobin, and the wide pulse (200 msec), longer than that of the dye laser, allows time for extensive diffusion of heat from the absorbing chromophores to the entire exposed field, generally resulting in nonselective alterations. Recent work (J. Finley, unpublished observations), however, suggests that at least in deeper zones of PWS *per se* there may be a measure of selectivity. It may be that the effectiveness of the argon laser in PWS with large abnormal blood-filled vessels, does relate, in part, to the hemoglobin content which might constitute the most significant chromophore mass [6]. Indeed, the concentration of energy in this area would certainly destroy the appropriate blood vessels.

It is quite likely nevertheless that the beneficial effects of the argon laser are a result of diffuse destruction of the upper dermis with its content of abnormal vessels and the establishment of new vessels with an entirely different flow pattern [12]. Selective destruction of the PWS vasculature by the dye laser, however, might be more effective therapeutically. It is important to recall, though, that chromophore content is the basis for the selective vascular necrosis. Pink PWS, the present challenge in therapy, have a limited erythrocyte content. Point vessel destruction in the network of these lesions probably would not significantly change the flow pattern. The purple lesions, on the other hand, already successfully treated with the argon laser, would present such a significant chromophore mass that the dye laser might be extremely effective with minimal destruction of tissue components other than vessels.

References

1. Solomon, H., Goldman, L., Henderson, B., et al. Histopathology of the laser treatment of port-wine lesions. J. Invest. Dermatol. 1968; 50:141–6.
2. Apfelberg, D., Maser, M., Lash, H. Argon laser management of cutaneous vascular deformities. West. J. Med. 1976; 124:99–101.
3. Apfelberg, D., Maser, M., Lash, H. Argon laser treatment of cutaneous vascular abnormalities. Ann. Plast. Surg. 1978; 1:14–8.
4. Apfelberg, D., Maser, M., Lash, H. Extended clinical use of the argon laser for cutaneous lesions. Arch. Dermatol. 1979; 115:719–21.
5. Apfelberg, D., Kosek, J., Maser, M., et al. Histopathology of portwine stains following argon laser treatment. Br. J. Plast. Surg. 1979; 32:232–7.
6. Noe, J., Barsky, S., Geer, D., et al. Portwine stains and the response to argon laser therapy: successful treatment and the predictive role of color, age and biopsy. Plast. Reconstr. Surg. 1980; 65:130–6.
7. Parrish, J. A. Photomedicine: potentials for lasers. In: Pratesi R, Sacchi, C. A., eds. Lasers in Photomedicine and Photobiology. Berlin/Heidelberg/New York: Springer-Verlag, 1980:2–22.
8. Anderson, R. R., Parrish, J. A. Optical properties of human skin. In: Regan, J. D., Parrish, J. A., eds. The Science of Photomedicine. New York: Plenum Press, 1982, pp.147–194.
9. Greenwald, J., Rosen, S., Anderson, R., et al. Comparative histological studies of the tunable dye (at 577 nm) laser and argon laser: the specific vascular effects of the dye laser. J. Invest. Dermatol. 1981; 77:305–10.
10. Dvorak, A., Mihm, M. C., Jr, Dvorak, H. Morphology of delayed-type hypersensitivity reactions in man. II. Ultrastructural alterations affecting the microvasculature and tissue mast cells. Lab. Invest. 1976; 34:179–91.
11. Moretti, G., Ellis, R., Mescon, H. Vascular patterns in the skin of the face. J. Invest. Dermatol. 1959; 33:103–12.
12. Finley, J., Barsky, S., Geer, D., et al. Healing of port wine stains after argon laser therapy. Arch. Dermatol. 1981; 117:486–9.

Cutaneous Laser Therapy: Principles and Methods
Edited by K. A. Arndt, J. M. Noe, and S. Rosen
© 1983 John Wiley & Sons Ltd

6

Differential Effects of Different Lasers on the Skin

Leon Goldman

Of the 12 laser systems used in science and medicine, the following nine systems have been used on human skin:

(1) ruby, normal mode, Q-switched, picoseconds,
(2) argon,
(3) CO_2,
(4) helium–neon,
(5) helium–cadmium,
(6) krypton,
(7) neodymium,
(8) neodymium YAG (Nd:YAG),
(9) ultraviolet.

The holmium, carbon monoxide, and the fluoride have not been used extensively.

In animal experimentation, the carbon monoxide (CO) and holmium lasers have also been used. Also, some operating probes have a combination of three lasers in the same attachment—CO_2, argon, and Nd:YAG. These probes are much more effective than some of the earlier designs where different laser systems were incorporated into a type of rotating drum, like a Gatling gun.

Many factors must be considered when studying the effects of lasers on the skin. Among the important variables are the irradiance (W/cm^2); the size, color, and other characteristics of the target area; and the pulse duration or speed with which the probe is passed over the skin with continuous wave (CW)

65

lasers. The effects of lasers on the skin have been observed and studied at many levels and by varying techniques: by gross inspection, color and color infrared photography, skin microscopy, replica mounts, scanning electron microscopy (SEM), routine histologic sections, electron microscopy, and with tissue culture techniques.

Are the different reactions in tissue only quantitative or qualitative? Investigators in China [1] as well as the United States [2] have been studying the effects of ultraviolet lasers on the skins. Despite the fact that the experiments for cancer were uncontrolled, these lasers do seem to offer possibilities in both investigative and clinical dermatology, particularly for selective effects on superficial blood vessels.

The ruby laser was the first to be studied for its effect on the skin because it was the first one available for clinical use. The cutaneous lesions it induced on normal skin were papules, erythema-edema, crusts, and deep thermocoagulation. For therapy of squamous cell carcinoma, energies as high as 20,000 J/cm^2 were used and deep necrosis was produced. The ruby laser was studied in normal mode, Q-switched, and for a few brief experiments in picosecond impacts.

When the Q-switched ruby laser (20–50 nsec) with energy densities of 2–4 J/cm^2 and power densities of 40–200 mW/cm^2 were used on tattoos, it caused immediate blanching and steam bubbles. This localized thermocoagulation necrosis, with minimal spread of heat through radiant and thermal conduction, left excellent cosmetic results.

Histological studies of the Q-switched and ruby lasers' impact showed that with low-power densities, there was transient blanching of tattoos. With moderate-power densities (200–300 mW/cm^2) s.e.m. studies showed cavernous structures about ink spots and no damage to epidermis or skin appendages. At about 300 mW/cm^2, there was damage to the epidermis [3]. The basic pathology was found to be thermocoagulation necrosis and the tissue reaction was similar to that of an electric burn. With 70–100 J/cm^2, relative resistance of the pilosebaceous unit and appendages was noted. This sparing of certain cutaneous structures allowed better cosmetic results but was of concern in the treatment of superficial spreading as well as of nodular melanoma. Low-output impacts of 20–30 J/cm^2 were also noted to cause bleaching of the hair. Scanning electron microscopy studies showed superficial topographic changes of wrinkling and slight scaling about the visible target area [4]. Picosecond impacts in one patient (the author) showed only localized reactions of thermocoagulation necrosis, with no dyskeratotic cells in the immediate area or in the superficial scar. With these short impacts, there was concern about soft X-rays developing in tissue.

The next system studied was the carbon dioxide (CO_2) laser. This laser could cause vaporization of the skin and could be used for photoexcision. A characteristic feature of its use was minimal bleeding with precise thermo-coagulation necrosis so that graft replacement could be achieved with no difficulty. We have observed this with excision of the angioma-like lesions of the blue rubber bleb nevus syndrome of the palms and face.

In contrast to the CO_2 laser, the Nd:YAG laser showed much more extensive thermocoagulation necrosis on liver tissue, but not on skin. The Nd:YAG laser of 300 W had been transmitted through a special quartz filter to the skin for treatment of tattoos and squamous cell carcinoma. Stokes [5] has pointed out that a 1.34-nm Nd:YAG laser, as opposed to the current 1.06-nm Nd:YAG laser, has greater penetration depth in animal tissue. He indicates that their laser is no substitute for the superficial photocoagulation of the argon laser, but would be useful chiefly for deep penetration. As yet, there are no clinical studies with this laser.

As the argon laser became used clinically, it was valued for its superficial effects on the skin with an almost selective effect on blood vessels. However, some superficial fibrosis was also evident. These data are discussed in greater detail elsewhere in this book.

In our laboratory, Greenberg and Tribbe [6] have used the pulsed organic dye laser for tissue transillumination studies. Test phantom models, but not skin, were studied using rhodamine 6G dye in the laser with a pulse output of 60 mJ. For clinical transillumination studies for early breast cancer detection, we have used low-output helium–neon, helium–cadmium, krypton, and Nd:YAG lasers.

We are sorely in need of controlled studies on the chronic effects of lasers on the skin. Only our clinical experience over the past two decades is available concerning chronic toxicity, and thus far there seem to be no harmful effects on the eye or the skin, for either patients or laser operators. Our investigative studies on chronic exposure have been only with the pulsed ruby laser (20 J/cm^2). Since initially used in 1962, no patients treated with the ruby laser have shown any evidence of carcinogenic effects.

The skin continues to offer a unique test model for study of the reactions of lasers on the tissues of humans. In brief, it parallels reactions in the eye and can be used to help understand not only the pathophysiology of laser reactions, but also to aid in the development of appropriate safety programs. Investigative work with laser systems in dermatology is important in basic photobiology, in photodiagnosis, and in use in clinical phototherapy.

References

1. Goldman, L. Laser dermatology in China. *Arch Dermatol.* 1981; **117**:566–8.

2. Anderson, R. R., Parrish, J. A. Microvasculature can be selectively damaging using dye lasers: a basic theory and experimental evidence in human skin. *Lasers in Surgery and Medicine.* 1981; **1**:268–76.
3. Ferguson, P. M., Paul, J. P., *et al.* Development of an out-patient technique for removing tattoos using a Q-switched pulsed ruby laser. Project Proposal, June 1980, Scottish Home and Health Department.
4. Goldman, L. *Applications of the Laser.* Cleveland: CRC Press, 1973:176.
5. Stokes, L. F. Biomedical utility of 1.34 Nd:YAG radiation trans. Personal communication.
6. Greenberg, D. B., Tribbe, M. D. Tissue diagnosis by laser transillumination and diaphanographic methods. In: Goldman, L., ed. *The Biomedical Laser. Technology and Clinical Applications.* New York: Springer-Verlag, 1981: 283–91.

SECTION III
Port Wine Stains

Cutaneous Lasery Therapy: Principles and Methods
Edited by K. A. Arndt, J. M. Noe, and S. Rosen
© 1983 John Wiley & Sons Ltd

7

History of Port Wine Stains

Robert M. Goldwyn

Although the nevus flammeus or capillary hemangioma (Figures 1 and 2) has been observed for centuries, it was not called port wine stain or port wine mark until after 1687, when he term 'port' first appeared in the English language [1]. Its origin was Oporto, the name of the chief city in Portugal from which the famous dark-red wine of that country was shipped. England's wars with Louis XIV led to the ban of French wines and an increased demand for 'red Portugal', also called port [2]. Evidence of the Englishman's preference for port is found in a reference to an incident that occurred in 1691: '314 English ships that went to Bordeaux and took in wine, and after sailed to port Oporto, and then came home, pretending it to be port' [1]. In English novels and in medical writings of the nineteenth century, 'port-wine stain' or 'port-wine mark' was frequently used to describe this common vascular anomaly: 'He has what is called a port-wine mark on the back of his neck' [1]. 'The hideous disfigurement of the countenance known as port-wine-mark which ordinarily colours the greater part of one side of the face of a dark moreen or purple-brown-red colour has long engaged my interest' [3].

Port wine stain is but another example of medicine's fondness for describing physical characteristics in terms of edibles, e.g. (grape, walnut, cherry) sized mass, nutmeg liver, and coffee ground material. Why medical terminology has such strong oral cathexis could well be the subject for discourse, not by a dermatologist or plastic surgeon but by a psychoanalyst.

As with any congenital anomaly, much superstition surrounds the port wine stain. These attitudes are reinforced by its striking color and its often prominent location. Among the laity, a common explanation for its origin is to implicate the mother—almost never the father—in some preterm trauma: the

71

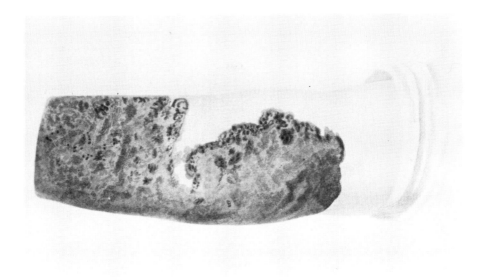

Figure 1   Nevus flammeus. (From Batemen, T. Delineations of cutaneous diseases exhibiting the characteristic appearance of the principal genera and species comprised in the classification of the late Dr. Willan; and completing the series of engravings begun by that author. London: Longman, 1817)

mother fell down the stairs or was frightened by a horse or ate strawberries or raspberries just before giving birth.

Until the advent of the laser, the port wine stain was treated by many techniques, single or multiple: partial or total excision with grafting, flap rotation, dermabrasion and grafting, cauterization, irradiation, obliteration by ligature, sclerosing agents, carbon dioxide snow, liquid nitrogen, cortisone, protamine, heparin locally and systemically, and, finally, visual reduction by tattoo and cosmetics [4]. The variety of these techniques attests to the inadequacy of the treatment.

Pooley [5], a physician in New York, compiled an extensive list of ways to remove the growth and to provide 'cosmetic treatment' as well as means for 'inducing atrophy' and for 'exciting inflammation in the tissue of the naevus', and thus obliterating its cells and vessels. He also mentioned 'an old woman's remedy': that of licking the tumor daily with the tongue. I presume that the patient and not the physician was supposed to do this.

Many of the treatments just enumerated succeeded by inducing the formation of scar tissue, a phenomenon that also occurs with laser therapy. To produce scarring and hopefully reduce vascularity, physicians in the past adopted unusual and hazardous measures. A frequent therapy was vaccination

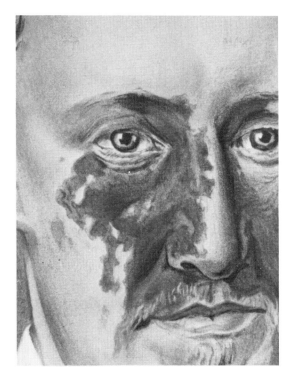

Figure 2   Nevus flammeus. (From Squire [3])

over and around the port wine stain. Another procedure was the injection of 'hospital pus'. These doctors had anticipated the value of recycling.

In 1876, Squire [3], an English physician, commented on the management of the port wine stain: 'I believe that no one who is affected with that misfortune ever applies for this particular grievance to any hospital for redress.'

Although the situation for the patient with this condition is much better now with the laser than before, problems remain. Then, as now, scarring can still be a complication. The therapeutic dilemma is that while some form of scar tissue seems necessary to improve the appearance of a port wine stain, too much is decidedly unwelcome.

No one with a sense of history expects that the laser in its present state is the ultimate treatment. While it is certainly more sophisticated and effective than licking the port wine stain, neverthelesss, it is not the end of our attempts to solve an extremely difficult problem. The eventual solution, whatever it is, will most likely be the result of the combined efforts of those in various disciplines of medicine, science, and industry.

References

1. *The Oxford English Dictionary*, Vol 7. Oxford: Clarendon Press, 1933: 1136–8.
2. Fletcher, W. *Port. An Introduction to its History and Delights*. London: Sotheby Parke Bernet, 1978:1–4.
3. Squire, A. J. B. *Essays on the Treatment of Skin Diseases. III. On port-wine mark and its obliteration without scar*. London: J & A Churchill, 1876.
4. Goldwyn, R. M., Rosoff, C. Cryosurgery for large hemangiomas in adults. *Plast. Reconstr. Surg.* 1969; **43**:605–11.
5. Pooley, J. H. Naevus. *New York Medical Journal*. 1873; **17**:593.

Cutaneous Laser Therapy: Principles and Methods
Edited by K. A. Arndt, J. M. Noe, and S. Rosen
© 1983 John Wiley & Sons Ltd

8

Clinical Syndromes Associated with Port Wine Stains

Robert S. Stern

Port wine stains (PWS), or nevus flammeus, most often occur as isolated cutaneous findings but may occur as part of syndromes that involve not only dermal blood vessels, but also those in other organs including abdominal viscera, bone, brain, and eye. In order to provide optimal care, the clinician must be aware of other findings possibly associated with the visible vascular lesion that was the cause of the patient's visit to the physician. Since syndromes which include PWS may require neurologic, ophthalmologic, or genetic evaluation, careful attention to associated signs and symptoms is particularly important. In addition, the clinician should remember that a PWS is only one type of vascular lesion seen at birth (see Chapter 15). In infants, the salmon patch and strawberry mark are more frequent and can easily be mistaken for the relatively uncommon PWS. Both have a better prognosis with respect to their ultimate cosmetic appearance and are not often associated with noncutaneous abnormalities.

Common vascular lesions of infancy

At birth and in early infancy, it may be difficult to distinguish between the three most common congenital vascular nevi of the skin—the salmon patch (nevus simplex), the strawberry mark, and the PWS (nevus flammeus). During infancy, the salmon patch is the most frequent vascular nevus. Seldom biopsied, this lesion's histopathology is not well defined. Its incidence varies substantially among ethnic groups. In Caucasions, the prevalence of these lesions may exceed 40 percent [1,2]. This lesion appears to be less common among Orientals and blacks [3]. The nape of the neck is the most frequent location for these lesions (80 percent), but they may also appear on the eyelids and glabella. Irrespective of site, these lesions usually fade away in the first year of life and require no therapy [4]. While some authors have suggested that they may be genetically determined lesions, salmon patches are not associated with noncutaneous abnormalities.

Strawberry marks are vascular hamartomas composed of both capillary and cavernous components. Estimates of the prevalence of strawberry marks vary greatly. Some authors suggest that up to 10 percent of infants manifest such lesions during the first year of life [5]. At birth, these lesions may be macular and resemble the salmon patch or PWS. According to maternal histories, less than one-third of strawberry marks are noted at birth, but more than 85 percent are noted in the first month of life [6]. Nearly all lesions cease to grow by one year of age [7]. The face and neck are the most frequent sites; the back and scalp are the next most frequent sites [6,7]. Their evolution to raised lesions typical of mixed capillary and cavernous hemangiomas and their subsequent involution distinguish these lesions from salmon patches and PWS.

Two large prospective studies demonstrate that most strawberry marks improve without therapy [6,7]. By the fifth year of life, half of all strawberry marks have resolved, and by the seventh year, over 70 percent show spontaneous resolution [6,7]. Lesions with the poorest prognosis are located on the mucous membrane of the lip or have failed to show any signs of regression by the end of the third year. Except for initiating rare thrombotic complications or obstructing a vital structure such as the eye, strawberry hemangiomas have little clinical or long-term significance other than their appearance. They rarely require treatment. Occasionally these lesions are very large, ulcerated, or obstruct vital structures. In such cases, therapy may be considered, and argon lasers have been used successfully in a few instance (see Chapter 17).

PWS have a far lower prevalence than salmon patches or strawberry marks. Jacobs and Walton estimate their frequency at 3 per 1000 [2]. Examination of 4600 newborn infants revealed only two with PWS [8]. Unlike the salmon patch, PWS do not spontaneously involute in infancy but slowly darken and, by adolescence, may become raised and have a cobblestone surface. The evolution of PWS is described in detail in Chapter 5. Hypertrophy of the subcutaneous tissue and bone underlying a PWS is not infrequent. While PWS can occur anywhere on the body, they are most frequently seen on the head and neck. Most often, PWS are isolated findings but they may be the cutaneous marker of a number of multisystem syndromes which include the following:

(1) Sturge–Weber syndrome,
(2) Klippel–Trenaunay–Weber syndrome,
(3) von Hippel–Lindau disease,
(4) Rubinstein–Taybi syndrome,
(5) Beckwith–Wiedemann syndrome,
(6) Cobb's syndrome,
(7) Coats' disease.

Sturge–Weber syndrome

In 1897, Sturge first described a patient with seizures and a PWS of the face. He hypothesized that the cause of this child's seizures was 'in all probability to be found in the presence of a port wine stain" on the surface of the brain' [9]. Sturge–Weber syndrome is a congenital disorder involving angiomatosis of the central nervous system, skin, and may include other organ systems such as the eye, oral pharynx, gastrointestinal tract, and bladder [10]. While usually sporadic, this disorder occasionally exhibits dominant inheritance. The PWS in the Sturge–Weber syndrome almost always occurs in the first division of the trigeminal nerve on the same side as the central nervous system angiomatosis (Figure 1). As a result of the angiomatosis of the meninges and other structures, abnormalities in the development of these structures occur. The most common central nervous system symptoms are seizures and mental retardation. In addition to vascular abnormalities, calcification of the brain may occur and is, in rare cases, bilateral [11]. Eye involvement occurs most often in patients with both upper and lower lid involvement [12]. Ophthalmologic abnormalities noted in this syndrome include choroid angiomas, eye enlargement, and congenital or acquired glaucoma. Angiomas of other organ systems, including bowel and kidney, bone, and gingiva, with subsequent bleeding risk and organ hypertrophy, have also been noted. The Sturge–Weber syndrome has been seen together with von Recklinghausen's disease (neurofibromatosis) and Klippel–Trenaunay–Weber disease [13]. Angiomatosis of the central nervous system indistinguishable from Sturge–Weber syndrome is occasionally seen without PWS being present [14].

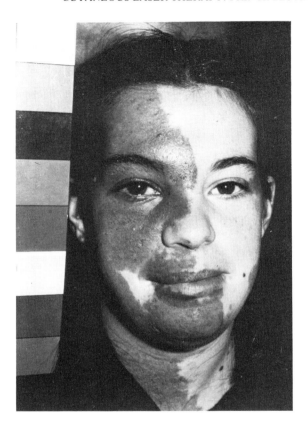

Figure 1   Port wine stain in patient with Sturge–Weber syndrome. Port wine stain
involves all divisions of trigeminal nerve

Klippel–Trenaunay–Weber syndrome

In 1900, Klippel and Trenaunay described a disorder characterized by PWS,
soft tissue and bony hypertrophy, and varicose veins [15]. These abnormalities occur most often on a single extremity or at times on ipsilateral upper and
lower extremities (Figure 2). The trunk and face may also be involved in this
usually unilateral disorder. Several investigators suggest the etiology of these
vascular deformities is a congenital malformation of the deep veins. In an
attempt to restore normal venous drainage of the affected limb, some authors
have recommended surgery but, even if successful, this has no effect on the
overlying PWS [16,17]. Radiographic evaluation may help identify patients
with vascular lesions most likely to be amenable to surgical intervention.
Urinary tract hemangiomas and rectal bleeding have been noted in patients

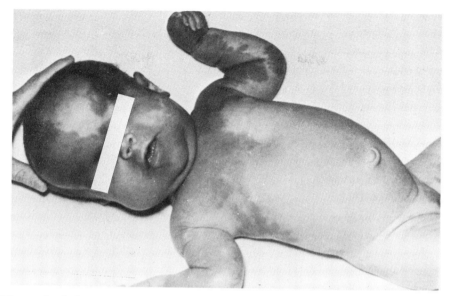

Figure 2   Infant with Sturge–Weber syndrome and Klippel–Trenaunay–Weber
syndrome with PWS of face and extremities

with Klippel–Trenaunay–Weber syndrome [16]. In addition to the superficial venous abnormalities seen in Klippel–Trenaunay–Weber syndrome, deep
vein varicosities of the limbs as well as pelvic veins often occur. The increased
blood flow resulting from these abnormalities is most probably responsible for
soft tissue and bony hypertrophy observed in such cases (Figure 3).

This disorder is usually evident at birth. Prenatal diagnosis of limb
hypertrophy by ultrasonography is possible [18]. Macrocephaly has been
seen in patients with Klippel–Trenaunay–Weber syndrome alone and in
combination with Sturge–Weber syndrome [19]. This disorder has also been
seen in association with tuberous sclerosis [20]. There is no evidence that
the PWS of Klippel–Trenaunay–Weber syndrome differ in their response to
argon laser therapy compared to PWS located in these areas but unassociated
with   the   underlying   bony   and   vascular   abnormalities   of   Klippel–Trenaunay–Weber syndrome.

von Hippel–Lindau syndrome

Von Hippel–Lindau syndrome is an inherited disorder which includes retinal
angiomatosis, angiomatosis of the central nervous system (especially involving
the cerebellum), as well as angiomas of the spinal cord, liver, and kidney. An
increased risk of renal cell carcinoma, as well as cysts of the pancreas, kidney,
and epididymis, and bilateral pheochromocytoma is present in patients with

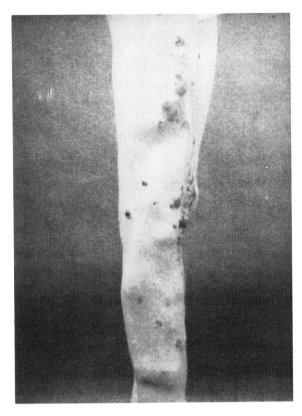

Figure 3   Varicosities of leg in a patient with Klippel–Trenaunay–Weber syndrome

von Hippel–Lindau syndrome. Port wine stains and other cutaneous hemangiomas only rarely have been reported as part of this syndrom [21]. Because it is
an autosomal dominant trait, and has a high risk of associated severe medical
complications, early recognition and appropriate genetic counseling is mandatory [22]. Ophthalmologic examination to identify the characteristic retinal
angiomatosis is the best screening examination to identify afflicted individuals.

Rubinstein–Taybi syndrome

In 1963, Rubinstein and Taybi described the syndrome of mental and motor
retardation, broad thumbs and broad first toes, growth retardation, microcephaly, ocular abnormalities, and failure of descent of the testes. In males,
cryptorchidism occurs frequently. Cutaneous abnormalities include PWS of the
forehead and nape of the neck (Figure 4). Hirsutism is occasionally noted.

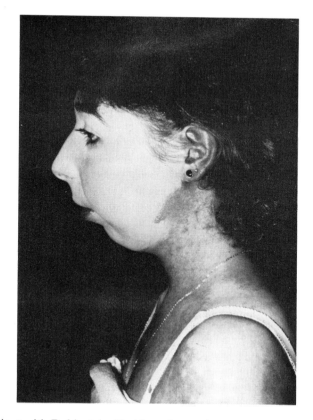

Figure 4   Patient with Rubinstein–Taybi syndrome demonstrating PWS of head and
neck and micrognathia

Pedigree analysis suggests autosomal recessive inheritance [23]. A case of
acute leukemia has been reported in a patient with Rubinstein–Taybi
syndrome, suggesting that this disorder might be included among those
genetically determined disorders associated with a higher risk of lymphoproli-
ferative diseases [24].

Beckwith–Wiedemann syndrome

The elements of the Beckwith–Wiedemann syndrome include defects in
closure of the abdominal wall, umbilical hernia and diastasis recti, viscerome-
galy, gigantism, advanced bone age, microcephaly, asymmetry, absence of
gonads, muscular hypertrophy, and diaphragmatic abnormalities. A PWS is
seen in a substantial fraction of these patients [25]. Immunodeficiency and
a higher risk of malignancy have also been reported in patients with this

disorder [25]. Pedigrees compatible with dominant, recessive, and sex-linked inheritance as well as sporadic cases have been reported [26]. Polyhydramnios is seen during half of pregnancies bearing infants with Beckwith–Wiedemann syndrome and the gigantism that accompanies this syndrome can be recognized by *in utero* ultrasound examination [27]. Metabolic abnormalities including hypoglycemia and hyperinsulinemia have been reported in affected infants [28]. The PWS seen in Beckwith–Wiedemann syndrome are indistinguishable from those occurring as isoalted cutaneous defects, but these patients are readily recognizable by their multiple developmental defects. The macroglossia and gigantism appear to be due to primary hyperplasia of muscles and other tissues rather than a reflection of hyperplasia secondary to increased circulation through abnormal blood vessels [29].

Cobb's syndrome

Cobb's syndrome is a rare disorder with fewer than 50 reported cases. Patients with this sporadic disorder have both cutaneous and meningiospinal angiomas. A PWS, angiokeratomas, or other vascular nevi are seen within two dermatomes of the area displaying spinal cord angiomatosis [30]. The size and type of cutaneous angioma may vary [31]. Symptoms associated with this syndrome are a result of the angioma's compression of the spinal cord. Renal angiomas, kyphoscoliosis, and angiomas of the vertebra can occur in Cobb's syndrome.

Coats' disease

Coats' disease consists of telangiectatic retinal vessels often seen in association with telangiectasia of the face, breasts, conjunctivae, and nailbeds [32]. A single case of a PWS in association with retinal telangiectasia and the absence of central nervous system involvement has been reported. This case may represent the chance occurrence of the sporadic PWS and the retinal abnormality of Coats' disease [32].

Miscellaneous syndromes

Apart from recognized syndromes, a variety of abnormalities have been reported in association with PWS. A family with dominantly inherited communicating hydrocephalus, posterior cerebellar agenesis, and PWS has been identified [33]. Cutis marmorata telangiectatica congenita (congenital livid network of the skin) has been reported in association with PWS and patent ductus arteriosis [34]. Port wine stains may occur more frequently in patients with Klinefelter's syndrome and trisomy 13 [35]. Vascular abnormalities of the skin are, however, present in only a small percentage of patients with these chromosomal disorders. Whether these findings represent only chance association of PWS with other abnormalities or distinct syndromes has not been established.

Proper care of patients with PWS requires special awareness of associated abnormalities, especially those involving the eye and central nervous system, which may not be apparent on initial examination.

References

1. Pratt, A. G. Birthmarks in infants. *Arch. Dermatol.* 1953; **67**:302–5.
2. Jacobs, A. H., Walton, R. G. The incidence of birthmarks in the neonate. *Pediatrics.* 1976; **58**:218–22.
3. Tan, K. L. Nevus flammeus of the nape, glabella and eyelids. *Clin. Pediatr.* 1972; **11**:112–8.
4. Smith, M. A., Manfield, P. A. The natural history of salmon patches in the first year of life. *Br. J. Dermatol.* 1962; **74**:31–3.
5. Bivings, L. Spontaneous regression of angiomas of children. *J. Pediatr.* 1954; **45**:643–7.
6. Simpson, J. R. Natural history of cavernous haemangiomata. *Lancet.* 1959; **2**:1057–9.
7. Bowers, R. E., Graham, E. A., Tomlinson, K. M. The natural history of strawberry nevus. *Arch. Dermatol.* 1960; **82**:667–79.
8. Alper, J., Holmes, L. B., Mihm, M. C., Jr. Birthmarks with serious medical significance: nevocellular nevi, sebaceous nevi, and multiple café-au-lait spots. *J. Pediatr.* 1979; **95**:696–700.
9. Sturge, W. A. A case of partial epilepsy apparently due to a lesion of the vaso-motor centres of the brain. Read to the Royal Society of Medicine. April 18, 1897.
10. Rook, A. Naevi and other developmental defects. In: Rook, A., Wilkinson, D. S., Ebling, F. J. G., eds. *Textbook of Dermatology.* Oxford: Blackwell, 1972: 146–7.
11. Boltshauser, E., Wilson, J., Hoare, R. D., Sturge–Weber syndrome with bilateral intracranial calcification. *J. Neurol. Neurosurg. Psychiatry.* 1976; **39**:429–35.
12. Barsky, S. H., Rosen, S., Geer, D. E., *et al.* The nature and evolution of port wine stains: a computer-assisted study. *J. Invest. Dermatol.* 1980; **74**:154–7.
13. Riley, F. C., Campbell, R. J. Double phakomatosis. *Arch. Ophthalmol.* 1979; **97**:518–20.
14. Lund, M. On epilepsy in Sturge–Weber disease. *Acta. Psychiatr. Neurol.* 1949; **24**:569–86.
15. Phillips, G. N., Gordon, D. N., Martin, E. C., *et al.* The Klippel–Trenaunay syndrome. Clinical and radiological aspects. *Radiology.* 1978; **128**:429–34.
16. Servelle, M., Bastin, R., Loygue, J., *et al.* Hematuria and rectal bleeding in the child with Klippel and Trenaunay syndrome. *Ann. Surg.* 1976; **183**:418–28.
17. Kinmonth, J. B., Young, A. E., Edwards, J. M., *et al.* Mixed vascular deformities of the lower limbs, with particular reference to lymphography and surgical treatment. *Br. J. Surg.* 1976; **63**:899–906.
18. Hatjis, C. G., Philip, A. C., Anderson, C. G., *et al.* The *in utero* ultrasonographic appearance of Klippel–Trenaunay–Weber syndrome. *Am. J. Obstet. Gynecol.* 1981; **139**:972–4.

19. Stephan, M. J., Hall, B. D., Smith, D. W., *et al.* Macrocephaly in association with unusual cutaneous angiomatosis. *J. Pediatr.* 1975; **87**:353–9.
20. Troost, B. T., Savino, P. J., Lozito, J. C. Tuberous sclerosis and Klippel–Trenaunay–Weber syndrome. *J. Neurol. Neurosurg. Psychiatry.* 1975; **38**:500–4.
21. Richards, R. D., Mebust, W. K., Schimke, R. N. A prospective study on von Hippel–Lindau disease. *J. Urol.* 1973; **110**:27–30.
22. Horton, W. A., Wong, V., Eldrich, R. von Hippel–Lindau disease. *Arch. intern. Med.* 1976; **136**:769–77.
23. Der Kaloustian, V. M., Afifi, A. K., Sinno, A. A., *et al.* The Rubinstein–Taybi syndrome. *Am. J. Dis. Child.* 1972; **124**:897–902.
24. Jonas, D. M., Heilbron, D. C., Albin, A. R. Rubinstein–Taybi syndrome and acute leukemia. *J. Pediatr.* 1978; **92**:851–2.
25. Sotelo-Avila, C., Gonzalez-Crussi, F., Fowler, J. W. Complete and incomplete forms of beckwith–Wiedemann syndrome: their oncogenic potential. *J. Pediatr.* 1980; **96**:47–50.
26. Lubinsky, M., Herrmann, J., Kosseff, A. L. Autosomal-dominant sex-dependent transmission of the Wiedemann–Beckwith syndrome. *Lancet.* 1974; **1**:932.
27. Weinstein, L., Anderson, C. *In utero* diagnosis of Beckwith–Wiedemann syndrome by ultrasound. *Radiology.* 1980; **134**:474.
28. Schiff, D., Colle, E., Wells, D., *et al.* Metabolic aspects of the Beckwith–Wiedemann syndrome. *J. Pediatr.* 1973; **82**:258–62.
29. Sokoloski, P. M., Ogle, R. G., Waite, D. E. Surgical correction of macroglossia in Beckwith–Wiedemann syndrome. *J. Oral. Surg.* 1978; **36**:212–5.
30. Jessen, R. T., Thompson, S., Smith, E. B. Cobb syndrome. *Arch. Dermatol.* 1977; **113**:1587–90.
31. Kissel, P., Dureux, J. B. Cobb syndrome. In: Vinken, P. J., Bruyn, G. W., eds. *Handbook of Clinical Neurology.* Vol. 14, *The Phakomatoses.* New York: American Elsevier, 1972:429–45.
32. Allen, H. B., Parlette, H. L. Coats' disease. *Arch. Dermatol.* 1973; **108**:413–5.
33. Nova, H. R. Familial communicating hydrocephalus, posterior cerebellar agenesis, mega cisterna magna, and port wine stain. *J. Neurosurg.* 1979; **51**:862–5.
34. Petrozzi, J. W., Rahn, E. K., Mofenson, H., *et al.* Cutis marmorata telangiectatica congenita. *Arch. Dermatol.* 1970; **101**:74–7.
35. Gupta, M. M., Grover, D. N. XXY Klinefelter's syndrome with bilateral cryptorchidism, obesity, multiple capillary hemangiomas and telangiectasia. *J. Urol.* 1978; **119**:143–4.

Cutaneous Laser Therapy: Principles and Methods
Edited by K. A. Arndt, J. M. Noe, and S. Rosen
© 1983 John Wiley & Sons Ltd

9

Nature and Evolution of Port Wine Stains

Seymour Rosen

Port wine stains (PWS) represent one type of congenital vascular malformation. These lesions are members of a larger group of congenital lesions termed nevus flammeus, which commonly involve the forehead, face, occiput, and nuchal regions and are present in 75 percent of newborns [1]. At birth, they are uniformly macular, pink to red, and most disappear by the end of the first year. PWS represent those nevi flammeus that continue into childhood and adult life. PWS can also be distinguished from other vascular lesions present in infancy and later life, among which are the strawberry nevus and arteriovenous malformation (see Chapter 15). Although initially he strawberry nevus may be similar to the PWS in appearance, eventually the strawberry nevus becomes raised, bulky, and compressible [2]. The most important distinction, however, is that the strawberry nevus undergoes a high rate of spontaneous involution, 70 percent by age 7 years, whereas the PWS does not disappear [2,3]. Histologically, the strawberry nevus is initially quite cellular with considerable capillary proliferation and the formation of predominately solid strands and masses. In older lesions, larger lumina are observed that are lined by flattened endothelium [4]. The arteriovenous malformation, uncommon in children, involves two distinct populations of vessels: thick-walled arteries and thin-walled veins [5]. Of all these lesions, the PWS alone is seen in association with the clinical conditions of glaucoma and the Sturge–Weber syndrome [6].

Because of studies suggesting that laser therapy might be an effective therapeutic modality, being beneficial in some but not all PWS [7–9], we decided to study biopsies from 100 patients with PWS. These studies [10] were intended to morphologically characterize the PWS lesion so that the pathophysiologic basis for present and future therapeutic modalities could be properly evaluated.

In an attempt to achieve as objective a characterization of PWS color as possible, two charts were prepared using material obtained from Letraset (Pantone graded color chart). One chart attempted to depict the normal flesh tones; the other included the PWS range (pink through purple). Each color was assigned a number and the numbers increased with deepening tone. A general assessment (percent) of facial involvement was made, and the face was arbitrarily divided into four quadrants (horizontal axis—canthus; vertical axis—midline) with the presence or absence of the PWS in each quadrant noted. Separate notations of eye (eyelid), nose, and lip, as well as neck, trunk, and extremity involvement were made. Patients were also evaluated as to the presence of glaucoma, epilepsy, and mental retardation.

The best oriented and prepared section from a 3-mm punch biopsy (see [10] for details) was chosen. Using a Wild M501 projection microscope (Heerbrugg), the following were quantitated: width and depth of biopsy; thickness of epidermis, papillary and reticular dermis, and subcutaneous tissue; number of hair follicles, sebaceous and sweat glands; degree (1 to 4) of hyperkeratosis, parakeratosis, melanin pigmentation, melanocytic proliferation, and elastosis. Since some patients had undergone previous tattoo treatment, the presence or absence of tattoo in the biopsy was recorded. The characteristics of each vessel in the subepidermal tissues were quantitated: dimensions (long and short axis), angulation (axis orientation: parallel to epidermis, 0°, 30°, 45°, 60°, or 90°), depth from dermal–epidermal junction (epidermal base was averaged into a straight line), presence or absence of erythrocytes, wall thickness, and degree of perivascular inflammation.

Initial studies indicated the difficulty in determining the demarcation between papillary and reticular dermis so analysis was facilitated by simply dividing the subepidermal tissue into 0.2-mm segments. For purposes of analysis, all vessel profiles were treated as ellipses. Computation of the following vessel parameters proved most useful: percent dermal area composed of vessels (vascular area); mean vessel area; mean wall thickness; vessel number; percent of vessels containing luminal erythrocytes (percent fullness); and mean vessel eccentricity (long/short axis). To maximize differences in vessel orientation, the degree of angulation was defined as the sum of the 60°- and 90°-oriented vessels divided by the total number of vessels minus those with 45° orientation. The data were both stored and analyzed as previously described [10]. Variation was expressed as standard deviation unless otherwise stated.

Clinical observations

The 100 PWS colors ranged from light pink to dark purple. The facial distribution of these lesions exhibited a wide range in the area involved, 25 ± 18 percent. Right-sided lesions were more common than left-sided, 58 *vs* 23 percent. The lesions involved two quadrants slightly more often than one, 47 *vs* 44 percent, but involvement of three or four quadrants occurred in a minority of cases, 3 and 6 percent, respectively. Involvement of eye, nose, lip, torso, and extremities was more comon in lesions having the greatest facial areas ($P < 0.001$). Eye involvement correlated with nose involvement ($P < 0.001$), but not with lip, neck, torso, or extremity. Nose involvement correlated with lip involvement ($P < 0.001$) but not with neck, torso, or extremity. The color of PWS did not correlate with facial area or quadrant distribution.

Histologic observations

Nonvessel parameters

The average biopsy's (Figures 1 and 2) width and depth was 2.38 ± 0.47 mm and 1.8 ± 0.42 mm, respectively. Epidermal thickness showed little variation (0.66 ± 0.0085 mm) in contrast to papillary dermal thickness (1.58 ± 0.125 mm) and reticular dermal thickness (1.37 ± 0.34 mm). Subcutaneous tissue was present in 69 percent of biopsies and measured 0.198 ± 0.23 mm. Number of hair follicles (1.96 ± 1.23), sebaceous glands (3.14 ± 2.23), and sweat glands (1.14 ± 0.92) varied widely. Hyperkeratosis (1.3 ± 0.5), parakeratosis (0 ± 0), melanin pigmentation (0.7 ± 0.5), and melanocytic proliferation (0.9 ± 0.4) had low values. The last two parameters, melanin pigmentation and melanocytic proliferation, correlated with each other ($P < 0.03$). Tattoo pigment was present in 8 percent of biopsies.

Vessel parameters

Mean vessel area and percent of vessels containing luminal erythrocytes (percent fullness) showed relative constancy, decreasing only moderately with depth (Figures 3 and 4). Each of these parameters exhibited a maximum at the 0.2–0.4 mm segment of dermis. In contrast, vessel number and percent dermal area composed of vessels (vascular area) decreased sharply with depth.

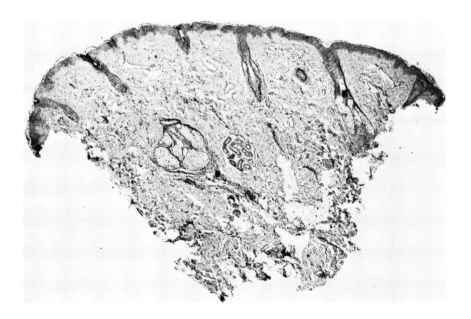

Figure 1   Skin biopsy from patient with port wine stain. This 11-year-old female had 2 percent vascular area, a mean vessel depth of 0.4 mm and a mean vessel area of 0.002 mm^2. ×42, hematoxylin & eosin

It should be noted that vascular area like mean vessel area, mean wall thickness, and percent fullness, was maximal at the 0.2–0.4 mm segment of dermis (Figure 3). Mean vessel eccentricity increased to a maximum at the 0.6–0.8 mm segment of dermis, then decreased; likewise, angulation increased then decreased with dermal depth, reaching maximum at the 0.4–0.6 mm dermal segment (Figure 3).

The lesions demonstrated a remarkable degree of internal consistency and homogeneity for most of their parameters (see [10] for details). Three parameters—mean vessel area, percent fullness, and mean wall thickness—exhibited good correlation between 0.2 mm increments in the first 0.8 mm of dermis. The vessel number and vascular area, which sharply decreased with depth, also had good internal correlations for the entire 1.0 mm dermal thickness. Vessel angulation maintained internal consistency for the entire dermis as well, but mean vessel eccentricity was an exception to all the previous histologic parameters in that it exhibited only weak homogeneity for the most superficial dermis and then no homogeneity at all. Hence, PWS exhibit homogeneity of vascular parameters uniformly throughout the first 0.8 mm of the lesion. The mean vessel depth of these lesions is 0.46 ± 0.17 mm, with a median depth of 0.31 mm.

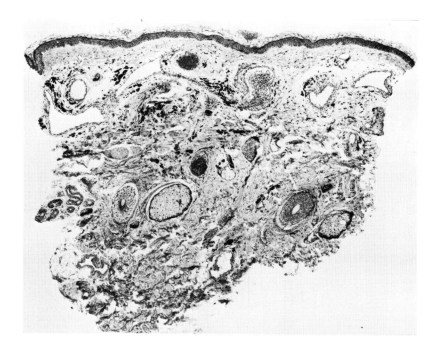

Figure 2   Skin biopsy from patient with port wine stain. This 29-year-old male, in contrast to the biopsy in Figure 1, had 6 percent vascular area, a mean vessel depth of 0.6 mm and a mean vessel area of 0.005 mm². ×42, hematoxylin & eosin. (From Barsky, S., Rosen, S., Geer, D., *et al*. The nature and evolution of port wine stains: a computer-assisted study. *J. Invest. Dermatol*. 1980; **74**:154–7. Copyright 1981, The Williams & Wilkins Company)

Different histologic parameters correlated with each other. Vascular area correlated strongly with mean vessel area (Figure 5) and percent fullness (Figure 6), but much less strongly with vessel number. Furthermore, mean vessel area and percent fullness correlated poorly with vessel number (Figure 7). Percent fullness, mean vessel area, and vascular area also exhibited minimal relationship to vessel depth and angulation, but inversely correlated with eccentricity.

Clinicopathologic correlations

Patient age ranged from 7 to 66 years with a mean of 26 ± 14. Vessel number, mean wall thickness, and mean vessel depth minimally increased with aging, but color substantially deepened (pink to purple) and vascular area and its correlates increased, with flat lesions becoming raised (Figure 8). The lesion's

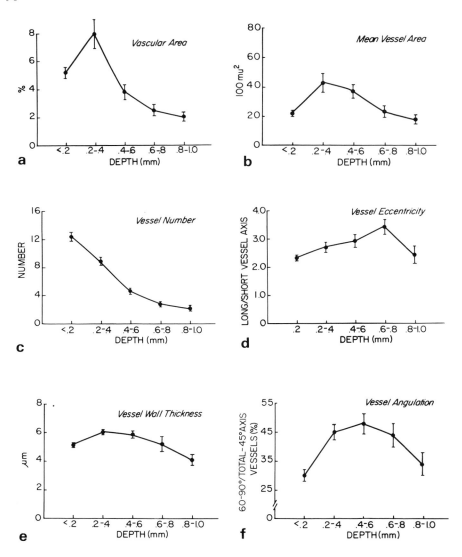

Figure 3   Relationship of various vessel measurements to increasing subepidermal depth. Both the percent of dermis occupied by vessels (vascular area) (a) and the mean vessel area (b) reach a peak 0.2–0.4 mm beneath the dermis. Vessel number (c) is highest just beneath the epidermis and then drops quickly. Vessel eccentricity (d) and wall thickness (e) show less variation with increasing depth; vessel angulation (f) peaks at 0.4–0.6 mm depth. Variation is expressed as standard error of the mean. (From Barsky, S., Rosen, S., Geer, D., *et al*. The nature and evolution of port wine stains: a computer-assisted study. *J. Invest. Dermatol.* 1980; **74**:154–7. Copyright 1981, The Williams & Wilkins Company)

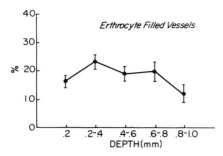

Figure 4   Relationship of erythrocyte-filled vessels (percent fullness) to depth. The percentage of vessels containing erythrocytes peaks (23.3 percent) 0.2–0.4 mm beneath the epidermis and falls to 11.6 percent at the 0.8–1.0 mm level. Variation is expressed as standard error of the mean

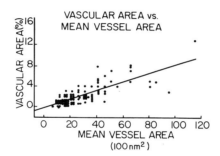

Figure 5   Relationship of percent of dermal area composed of vessels (vascular area) to mean vessel area. As would be expected, there is a strong relationship (Pearson correlation coefficient 0.79) between these two parameters. (From Barsky, S., Rosen, S., Geer, D., et al. The nature and evolution of port wine stains: a computer-assisted study. *J. Invest. Dermatol.* 1980; **74**:154–7. Copyright 1981, The Williams & Wilkins Company)

facial area did not change with age, but age correlated with the degree of elastosis ($P < 0.02$).

Lesion color strongly correlated with histologic parameters, percent fullness, vascular area, and mean vessel area, but correlated poorly with vessel number, mean vessel depth, and other histologic indices. Facial area and quadrant distribution were independent of any histologic parameter.

Glaucoma occurred in 10 percent of patients (mean age 21 ± 7 years). Every patient with glaucoma had eye (eyelid) involvement as well as superior and inferior quadrant involvement on the side affected with glaucoma. Twenty-seven patients (mean age 24 ± 13 years) demonstrated similar distribution of their PWS, superior and inferior quadrant and eye involvement, but no glaucoma. Mental retardation was seen in 5 percent of patients and all of these had glaucoma. The groups with glaucoma and mental retardation showed no difference in color or any histologic parameter, but differed markedly in

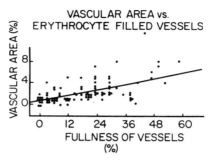

Figure 6   Relationship and percent of dermal area composed of vessels (vascular area) to erythrocyte-filled vessels (percent fullness). There is a strong correlation (Pearson correlation coefficient 0.60) between vascular area and percent fullness. The relationship between vascular area and vessel number is less impressive (Pearson correlation coefficient 0.37)

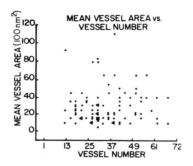

Figure 7   Relationship of mean vessel area and vessel number. The lack of relationship between mean vessel area and vessel number (Pearson coefficient 0.0024), and the very strong correlation between mean vessel area and percent dermal area composed of vessels (vascular area) shown in Figure 5, indicates that the most significant determinant of vascular area is mean vessel area rather than number of vessels

facial area and quadrant involvement compared to the patients lacking these associated conditions. Patients with mental retardation had a mean facial area of 69 ± 23 percent and patients with glaucoma had a mean facial area of 56 ± 26 percent compared to 22 ± 14 percent lacking these conditions; both differences were significant ($P < 0.001$). All but one patient with mental retardation had three- or four-quadrant involvement.

Discussion

Because of recent observations that argon laser therapy was beneficial in some PWS, the question of efficacy of biopsy as a predictor of response was raised.

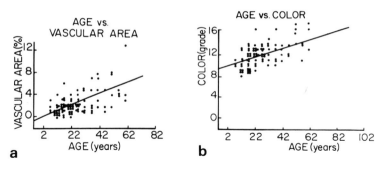

Figure 8 Relationship of age to percent of dermal area composed of vessels (vascular area) (a) and color (b). As age increases so does vascular area (Pearson correlation coefficient 0.63). There is an equally good relationship between age and deepening color (pink to purple) (Pearson correlation coefficient 0.60). (From Barsky, S., Rosen, S., Geer, D., *et al.* The nature and evolution of port wine stains: a computer-assisted study. *J. Invest. Dermatol.* 1980; **74**:154–7. Copyright 1981, The Williams & Wilkins Company)

Previous studies had demonstrated that laser radiation is preferentially absorbed by pigment, and that the argon laser specifically interacts with hemoglobin and its derivatives [7,11,12]. Because of this dependence on chromophore occurrence and its dispersion within tissues, it was felt that only a detailed structural analysis of the biopsy could produce predictive factors for laser therapy response. It soon became clear that nowhere in the literature had vascular lesions been analyzed from the standpoint of their spatial relationships, either at one point in time or from an evolutionary standpoint. The use of this computer-assisted structural analysis allowed us to realize observations and characteristics of the lesions that were not possible by simple inspection. The variation noted in some PWS also was a limiting factor. However, a representative area was biopsied and our patient population was large. Biopsies from normal facial skin would have been useful as controls in the evaluation of data; however, such facial biopsies could not be justified.

The central abnormalities characterizing PWS appear to be an increase in both vessel number and ectasia compared to normal skin, but each of these parameters and their correlates exhibit different properties. Vessel number sharply decreases with depth with the majority of vessels located in the immediate subepidermal dermis. In contrast, mean vessel area exhibits a lesser degree of variation throughout the dermis and achieves a maximum at the 0.2–0.4 mm segment. Hence PWS in respect to vessel number are superficial lesions, but in respect to vessel ectasia, involve the vessels throughout their skin thickness. It is important to recognize in the present study that vascular profiles are equated with vessel number and that a single racemose vessel might be considered as multiple distinct vessels in a histologic section. Indeed, since there was poor correlation between aging and vessel number, we feel that the

PWS probably represents a progressive ectasia and aneurysmal dilatation of a cutaneous vascular plexus that was normal at one stage of its development, i.e. *no true increase in vessel number*. Such a hypothesis is consistent with the observations of Miescher [3] and Schnyder [13] that abnormalities in histologic sections of nevus flameus in infancy or early childhood are minimal. Winkelmann *et al.*'s findings [14] in histochemical preparations are also in concert with this possibility: 'In nevus flammeus, blind sacs project from the wall of the capillary in many directions and constitute perhaps the basic pathologic finding of this vascular nevus.'

Histologic characteristics of the PWS, in general, exhibit strong layer-to-layer correlation throughout the entire lesion's thickness. This indicates that although these parameters change with depth, they exhibit a homogeneity in that change. Thus the PWS has to be viewed as an 'ordered' lesion, composed of a cluster of vessels, not in a haphazard arrangement, but one with a characteristic architecture. Furthermore, this 'ordered' lesion evolves in an orderly and characteristic manner. Vessel number and mean vessel depth correlate poorly with age, while mean vessel area, vascular area, and percent fullness all increase with age. These observations are consistent with previous observations that PWS darken with advancing age [13,15], and that prominent ectasia is characteristic of the adult PWS [13]. It should be pointed out that this correlation is not perfect; that the rate of ectasia varies from patient to patient; that 'older' patients may still have a much 'younger' lesion and young patients may have an 'aged' PWS. The reasons for this progressive ectasia and for the varying rates of ectasia are unknown. We feel that one explanation might be that the colagen degeneration that accompanies age may weaken the supporting dermal structures and allow the abnormal vessels to dilate. At the same time, tissue perfusion pressure increases with age. Indeed, our studies have demonstrated that mean vessel area does correlate with elastosis ($P < 0.01$), but since both these parameters increase with age, this relationship is less meaningful. Elastosis cannot be the only factor in this progressive ectasia since there are cases in our series in which the patients are old, their mean vessel area is high, but there is minimal concomitant elastosis.

No histologic parameter or lesion color distinguishes patients with glaucoma or Sturge–Weber syndrome. Their lesions seem identical to PWS without associated abnormalities. The fundamental difference between these groups lies in the extent of lesion and quadrant distribution, i.e. the facial percentage in glaucoma and Sturge–Weber cases is much greater than in uninvolved patients. This observation would seem reasonable since the more extensive the field of vascular abnormality, the great chance that vessels near the optic nerve and leptomeninges would be involved. Indeed, every patient with glaucoma had both superior and inferior quadrant involvement, a finding in agreement with other studies that relate the occurrence of glaucoma in PWS to involvement of both first and second divisions of the trigeminal nerve

[16,17]. Hence, it is location and extent of abnormality that determines the incidence of glaucoma.

In essence, therefore, the central abnormalities characterizing PWS are an apparent increase in vessel number and ectasia. Vessel number is highest in the immediate subepidermal area and then rapidly diminishes; mean vessel depth is 0.46 ± 0.17 mm. In contrast, mean vessel area shows less variation throughout the dermis, ectatic vessels being present when vessel number is very low. The product of both factors determines the percent of dermis occupied by vessels, but the mean vessel area is the major determinant. While age correlates poorly with vessel number, it correlates well with both progressive vessel ectasia and color shifts (pink to purple). Furthermore, this lack of correlation between aging and vessel number suggests that PWS is not a vascular proliferative lesion (hemangioma) but a progressive dilatation and ectasia of the superficial vascular plexus. Each of the multiple vessel parameters analyzed (vessel number, mean vessel area, wall thickness, angulation, and luminal erythrocyte content) exhibited strong layer-to-layer correlation within the first 0.8 mm of tissue beneath the epidermis, indicating homogeneity of vessel characteristics within the lesion. The size of the lesion and facial quadrant distribution do not change with age nor are they related to any histologic parameters. However, patients with glaucoma and mental retardation have more extensive facial involvement than individuals without these findings.

References

1. Caro, W. H. Tumors of the skin. In: Moschella, S., Pillsbury, D., Hurley, H., eds. *Dermatology*. Philadelphia: WB Saunders Co, 1975:1323–1406.
2. Bowers, R. E., Graham, E., Tomlinson, K. The natural history of the strawberry nevus. *Arch. Dermatol.* 1960; **82**:59–72.
3. Miescher, G. Uber plane Angiome (Naevi hyperaemici). *Dermatologica*. 1953; **106**:176–83.
4. Montgomery, H. *Dermatopathology*. New York: Harper & Row, 1967:1096.
5. Girard, C., Graham, J., Johnson, W. Arteriovenous hemangioma (arteriovenous shunt). A clinicopathological and histochemical study. *J. Cutan. Pathol.* 1974; **1**:73–87.
6. Koblenzer, P. J., Koblenzer, C. S. Anomalies of the vascular system as they affect the skin. *Clin. Pediatr.* 1966; **5**:95–102.
7. Apfelberg, D. B., Morton, R., Lash, H. Argon laser treatment of cutaneous vascular abnormalities: progress report. *Ann. Plast. Surg.* 1978; **1**:14–8.
8. Ginsbach, G., Hohler, H., Lemperle, G. Treatment of hemangiomas with argon laser (abstr). *Plat. Reconstr. Surg.* 1978; **62**:145.
9. Ohmori, S. Effect of argon laser beam upon port wine stain (abstr). *Plastic Surgery Forum*. 1978; **1**:56.
10. Barsky, S., Rosen, S., Geer, D., *et al.* The nature and evolution of port wine stains: a computer-assisted study. *J. Invest. Dermatol.* 1980; **74**:154–7.

11. Goldman, L., Rockwell, R. J. *Lasers in Medicine*. New York: Gordon and Breach, 1971:163–211.
12. Solomon, H., Goldman, L., Henderson, B., *et al*. Histopathology of the laser treatment of port-wine lesions. *J. Invest. Dermatol*. 1968; **50**:141–6.
13. Schnyder, U. W. Zur Klinik und Histologie der Angiome. 2. Mitteilung: die Feuermaier (Naevi teleangiectatici). *Arch. Dermatol. Syphilol. (Berlin)*. 1954; **198**:51–74.
14. Winkelmann, R. K., Scheen, R. S., Pyka, R. A., *et al*. Cutaneous vascular patterns in studies with injection preparation and alkaline phosphatase reaction. In: Montagna, W., Ellis, R. A., eds. *Advances in Biology of Skin*. Vol. 2. New York: Pergamon Press, 1961:1–137.
15. Reed, R. J., O'Quinn, S. Vascular neoplasms. In: Fitzpatrick, T. B., Arndt, K. A., Clark, W. H., Jr, *et al*., eds. *Dermatology in General Medicine*. New York: McGraw-Hill Book Co, 1971:533–49.
16. Stevenson, R. F., Morin, J. D. Ocular findings in nevus flammeus. *Can. J. Ophthalmol*. 1975; **10**:136–9.
17. Stevenson, R. F., Thomson, H. G., Morin, J. D. Unrecognized ocular problems associated with port wine stain of the face in children. *Can. Med. Assoc. J*. 1974; **111**:953–4.

Cutaneous Laser Therapy: Principles and Methods
Edited by K. A. Arndt, J. M. Noe, and S. Rosen
© 1983 John Wiley & Sons Ltd

10

Predictive Value of Age, Color, and Biopsy on Argon Laser Therapy of Port Wine Stains

Joel M. Noe

Port wine stains (PWS) most commonly appear on the face and neck. Studies to date have shown an incidence of less than 1 percent, which may understate the true incidence for a number of reasons [1,2]. Frequently parents have stated that the PWS was not visible at birth. Given the relative anemic state and the relative erythematous condition of the skin of the infant, one can understand how a PWS may not be appreciated at the time of birth, thus understating any studies based on birth records or physical examination at birth. The color of the PWS is stable in certain patients, while in others it changes, darkening with time. The major histologic problems seen are an inceased flow and a progressive ectasia of the superficial dermal vessels [3]. Associated with these changes is a darkening of the color from pink to red to purple and an elevation of the surface from smooth to irregular to the 'cobblestone' pattern seen in the older patient with a purple PWS.

Cosmetics are the mainstay for the treatment of PWS in the United States. However, when the PWS has a darker color, thicker, more unnatural-appearing cosmetics must be used. Also, when the PWS is associated with hypertrophy or elevation of the skin, makeup tends to accentuate the lesion rather than mask it. The daily use of cosmetics is very time-consuming and expensive. There is always the risk of allergic and sensitivity reactions and dependency. Other treatment methods besides the laser have been tried, but have not withstood the test of time. For very small PWS, an excision with a primary closure may be useful. Skin grafts incur the price of a donor-site scar and provide skin that usually is not a good color match for the facial skin. In addition, when compared with the changes in facial color effected by emotion, disease, and the seasons, the skin graft remains a fixed unalterable color.

Current state of the art

The argon laser is the method of choice for treating PWS at the present time. However, while most of the literature states that the argon laser produces a monochromatic, coherent, collimated light that is selectively absorbed by hemoglobin, this is overly simplistic. In fact, the argon laser has six different wavelengths ranging from 457.9 to 514.5 nm [4–6]. It is not monochromatic. The two peak wavelengths are 488 nm and 514.5 nm and account for over 80 percent of the argon laser energy output. Simply put, the argon laser is useful when treating PWS because the blue-green light is preferentially absorbed by the oxygenated hemoglobin in superficial dermal ectatic vessels. The light energy is transformed to heat and heat damage ensues, vessels thrombose, and the PWS lightens. In reality, however, the skin is neither an ideal optical medium nor are the present argon laser machines able to deliver a light that is selectively absorbed by just the hemoglobin molecules [7]. The very interaction of argon laser radiation and oxygenated hemoglobin is not fully understood.

Regardless, good results, defined by marked lightening and flattening without scarring, are obtained with the present argon laser treatment. The full potential of the argon laser has not as yet been tested because of the limitations imposed upon us by our inadequate knowledge of the basic mechanism of action as well as the limitations imposed by the present status of the machines. The machines used are essentially first-generation devices. We have a choice of paths to follow. On the one hand we can attempt to improve the machine and its use; for example, decrease pulse duration, increase power, increase monochromaticity, and thereby hope to make it more selective. Another approach would be to make the ectatic vessels and their contents more absorbent at the same time that the surrounding tissues are made less absorbent. The freezing techniques of Gilchrest et al. [8] show promise in this regard. A third alternative might be a combination of spectroscopy—by elucidating the actual peak absorption wavelength of the PWS—and use of the tunable dye laser to match it [9] (see Chaps. 3 & 5).

Predictive role of color, age, and biopsy

A study was done with 62 Caucasian patients with PWS on their face and neck [10]. Prior to argon laser treatment, 3-mm punch biopsies were obtained from a representative region of the lesion. Patients then received treatment to a 2-cm diameter test circle with the blue-green argon laser (Coherent Radiation model 1000). The test patch was adjacent to the site of this biopsy. Each patient ws treated identically: the irradiance was 255 W/cm^2 with a 0.1-cm diameter cirular spot, a pulse duration of 0.2 sec, and an energy fluence of 51 J/cm^2. Patients were then evaluated approximately 4 months later. The color of the test circle after treatment was noted, compared to the pretreatment color, and the color shift determined. The occurrence of scarring and the color shift were combined in an overall assessment of the lesion's response to laser therapy. A desirable result occurred in 73 percent of patients; an undesirable result in 27 percent, with an 11 percent incidence of hypertrophic scarring (see Table 1). Response ws predicted with varying degrees of accuracy with regard to the result of the test patch: the age of the patient, the color of the lesion, and the vascular parameters, especially percent 'fullness' (amount of hemoglobin present in the vessels), contributed to the response.

Color of lesion

The spectrum of PWS colors tends to go from pink to red to purple. Pink lesions are most easily covered by makeup. Purple lesions, because of their darker color and because of their frequent association with hypertrophy and vascular nodules, are most difficult to cover with cosmetics. Fortunately, there is a much bigger difference, and hence improvement, between the purple lesion pretreatment and the lighter color post-treatment when compared to the pink lesion pretreatment and the color post-treatment (see Figure 1); and, it is the older patients who have the darker lesions. The results of the above study show that the darker the lesion, the greater the degree of lightening and the less the incidence of scarring. Obversely, the ligher the lesion, the less the degree of lightening and the greater the incidence of scarring.

Age of the patient

It can be seen from Table 1 that the older the patient, the better the result. There are a number of reasons for this. As a patient ages, PWS color gets darker. As noted above, the darker colors and associated elevations of the lesions make them amenable to greater improvement. The vessels are more

Table 1   Analysis of factors determining response to argon laser therapy

	Desirable*	Undesirable*	Scarring*†
Age (years)			
< 17	5	7	3
≥17 < 37	24	10	3
≥ 37	16	0	1
Color (graded units)			
Pink (8–9)	1	8	4
Red (10–13)	20	9	2
Purple (≥ 14)	24	0	1
Vascular area (%)			
< 2	0	8	2
≥ 2 < 5	11	6	3
≥ 5	34	3	2
Mean vessel area (100 μm²)			
<15	4	10	3
15 < 25	11	6	2
≥ 25	30	1	2
Fullness (%)			
≤ 3	0	12	6
> 3 < 15	10	5	0
≥ 15	35	0	1

*Indicates number of patients.
†This group of patients is a subset of those noted under 'Undesirable'.
Source: Noe, J. M., Barsky, S. H., Geer, D. E., *et al.* Port wine stains and the response to argon laser therapy: successful treatment and the predictive role of color, age and biopsy. *Plast. Reconstr. Surg.* 1980; **65**:130–6.

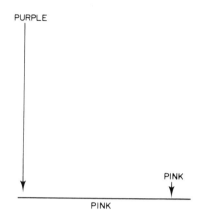

Figure 1   There is a much bigger difference, and hence improvement, between the purple lesion pretreatment and the lighter color post-treatment when compared to the pink lesion pretreatment and the color post-treatment

ectatic with more hemoglobin present. In addition, older people tend to scar less than younger people with the same degree of trauma.

Psychologically it is the young patients who stand to benefit most from removing a blemish from their face [11]. However, because of the increased incidence of scarring, especially in those patients with the lighter-colored lesions, the risk of the procedure is greater. The older patient, with the purple lesion, with the elevated lesion, with vessels full of red blood cells, tends to scar less. Local anesthesia is easier to apply and psychologically less stressful to a mature adult when compared to an immature child. Hence, the younger patient is more likely to need general anesthesia with its attendant costs and risks.

Histologic criteria

In the papillary dermis is an increased number of vessels that are stable in number, but become progressively ectatic over time [3,12–14]. It was initially thought that the red color of the oxygenated hemoglobin molecules in these vessels would selectively absorb the blue-green light of the argon laser. However, because of the optical qualities of the skin, the different wavelengths of the argon laser, and the nature of the PWS, the reaction between argon light and the skin is not as specific as originally thought. Argon light selectively affects vessels less than 0.5 mm in diameter that lie within the upper 1.5 mm of dermis, with a relative sparing of skin appendages—a major distinguishing factor between pure thermal burns and laser reactions. As patients age, greater ectasia is found in PWS with an associated increased number of red blood cells in the vessels. There are different categories of PWS noted on the basis of the size and the level of the affected vessels [15].

Initially, a 3-mm punch biopsy was obtained from each patient, as was done in the study cited above. The data showed that a number of factors histologically were predictive of ultimate results (see Table 1). The fuller the vessel was with red blood cells, the larger the vessel, the more superficial the vessel, the better the result. These results correlated with the color of the lesion and the age of the patient. The results of these initial and other studies were such that no longer are biopsies needed on the majority of the patients. In certain patients, other factors noted above (e.g. color of lesion, age of patient) correlate so well with the data obtained in biopsies that they can be used independently to predict final results. The technique used to obtain the biopsy is to select an area of the PWS that is representative of the whole area. Two percent Xylocaine is used. A 2-mm punch biopsy is obtained and the resultant wound is closed with a single stitch. The results are analyzed by the methods of Barsky, Rosen, and Finley [3,10,12]. The biopsy data are especially helpful in the 'borderline' PWS, e.g. younger ages, lighter colors, or when all the other factors prove indeterminate.

Test patch

A *test patch* is performed in an area 2 cm in diameter that is representative of the whole PWS and visible to the patient, but not necessarily in the central part of the face. Avoiding the central part of the face limits the inconvenience associated with the dressing required after treatment. The advantages of a test patch are multiple. It allows the patient to decide whether or not to continue treatment—on the basis of lightening, degree of depression, presence or absence of scarring—before obligating himself/herself to treatment of the whole area. Also, the patient can experience the costs and discomfort of the healing, the dressings, the wound care required, and the possible time lost from work. Four months later the test patch is evaluated. For the majority of patients this period of time is required before assessment of the degree of lightening and the presence or absence of scarring can be made. A few patients have taken as long as a year, and others have taken as short a period as 6 weeks, but these have been in the minority. The physician and the laser team can also assess the response to laser therapy on the basis of the test patch, as well as the patient's response to this degree of lightening.

One limitation of the test patch is that, due to its location on the periphery of the face, the incidence of scarring is less than that experienced on the central part of the face. In addition, the test patch is limited to the extent that the PWS is not homogeneous. Oftentimes one will see different colors in different areas of the same face, and to this extent one test patch has its limitations. On occasion more than one test patch has been found to be useful to the patient. When evaluating the test patch one must beware of the illusion created by evaluating a test patch surrounded by untreated PWS and then comparing that to treated PWS bordered by normal facial skin (N. A. Gilchrest, personal communication).

Technique

An initial consultation is held with the patient and family [16]. The alternative methods of treatment, the expected results, the limitations, the risks and complications, both short and long term, are presented. The patient is fully informed. Photographs are taken.

Local anesthesia is used. Two percent Xylocaine without epinephrine is injected in the deep dermal–subcutaneous level [17]. This may maximally vasodilate the vessels and thus provide a larger 'target' area. Field blocks have not been found to be useful.

All procedures are done on an ambulatory basis. When larger areas are done the work proceeds from the periphery to the central part of the face. Usually a 5 cm × 5 cm area is done at each session. The area treated is a function of the size and location of the PWS, as well as of such practical considerations as acceptance by the patient of wounds and dressings at the workplace and in other daily life activities.

Treatment and wound care advice is given both verbally and in writing (see Table 2) [18]. Oftentimes patients and their families are quite anxious and, hence, appreciate the written instructions to take home. The information provided explains what to expect following laser therapy as well as how to care for the treated area. The wound tends to weep for 1–3 weeks after treatment, at which time the weeping stops and/or a scab forms. The amount of pain noted is quite minimal. Marked swelling of the eyelids usually occurs when they or the periorbital area are treated. This swelling responds well to ice placed on the lids as well as head elevation plus forceful winking. The wound care advice is aimed at keeping the area clean. Soap and water is the simplest and best way to achieve this. The wound should be healed prior to the application of any cosmetics. Scabs are best left intact and should be allowed to fall off on their own. Prior to the next treatment, the patient is asked not to get a sunburn in the area to be treated; the erythema produced may minimize the absorption of the argon laser by the hemangioma. The patient is asked to avoid aspirin or aspirin-containing compounds to minimize any bleeding at the time of treatment.

Laser application: the physician is seated next to the patient with his hands stabilized and holding the laser fiberoptic unit about 2 inches from the skin. The machine (Coherent Radiation Dermatologic Model 1000) control module power reading is confirmed by an independent meter. A pulse duration of 0.2 sec is used with a maximum repetition rate; 1.2–1.5 W is used for the remaining parts of the face and the darker lesions, especially those associated with hypertrophy. When blanching is noted, the light beam is moved.

The upper lip and circumoral area are treated last to take advantage of the knowledge gained in a particular patient with regard to the ideal power necessary to obtain blanching and the type of healing noted in the earlier areas. It is not known why this area is most commonly subject to scarring. Anecdotally, pressure on the area, the 'stripping' technique, immobilization of the area, and application of topical steroids to inhibit collagen synthesis have all been used, but without any as yet documented evidence of value.

Evaluation results

In all studies the majority of patients have noted a favorable response to argon laser treatment defined by marked lightening without scarring [10,15,18–23] (see also Chapter 11). However, I believe there has been an obsession with color changes and the presence or absence of scarring with a neglect of other factors. The lightening of the color and the *flattening of the lesion* usually permit the patient to use more natural-appearing, less expensive, and more quickly applied cosmetics. Oftentimes there is less need for any

Table 2   Care following laser treatment

What to expect after laser treatment:
- In the first few weeks the treated skin may 'weep' and then a scab may form. Some people will heal without forming a scab.
- After the scab falls off, the treated area may look red. This is *expected*. It *does not* mean that the treatment did not work.
- The local anesthetic, Xylocaine, plus the laser treatment may leave the treated area swollen for the next several hours or even days. If the area treated was near your eyes, your eyelids may become swollen.
- It may take from two (2) to nine (9) months for this area to lighten in color. Once this process has begun, the skin color will continue to lighten for the next year.

How to care for your treated area:
Swelling
- Sleep with your head elevated on several pillows to decrease facial swelling.
- Ice may decrease swelling of your eyelids if used soon after treatment and for 24 hours thereafter.
- Forced 'winking' of your eyes helps decrease swelling in eyelid muscles.
- An eye patch may be worn for several days.

Skin care until 'weeping' stops and/or a scab forms
- Wash the area gently three (3) times a day with Dial soap and rinse well with water.
- Gently pat dry and apply a thin layer of Bacitracin ointment over the area.
- After each washing, cover the area with a clean Telfa dressing or plastic strips (such as Band-Aids).
  (*Note*: Remove dressings carefully. Do not pull the dressing off if it is sticking to the area. Instead—soak the dressing in water until it comes off easily.)

Skin care after 'weeping' stops and/or scab forms
- Use soap and water. Bacitracin dressings are no longer necessary.
- You may apply makeup on the treated area only *after* the scab has *fallen off*, which may take two (2) weeks. However, waiting to apply makeup reduces the risk of infection.
- When the area is completely healed (which may take up to three (3) weeks), you may resume shaving.
- You may swim in clean water. Remember to wash with soap and water after swimming.

What to avoid before and after laser treatment:
Avoid direct sun exposure
- Treated skin may be overly sensitive to the sun. The laser-treated area should not be exposed directly to the sun for ten (10) weeks after treatment. A sunscreen containing PABA is recommended.
- Avoid direct sun exposure to any area of skin that will be treated with laser for three (3) weeks prior to the treatment. Sunburn, which causes redness of the superficial skin, may absorb the laser light and thereby decrease the effectiveness of the treatment.
- In order to evaluate the laser's effectiveness, your skin must not be sunburned. Avoid direct sun exposure to the treated area for three (3) weeks before an evaluation visit.

Avoid aspirin products before treatments
- Aspirin or aspirin-containing products (Bufferin, Anacin, Excedrin, Dristan, etc.) *must* be avoided for seven (7) days before your next treatment. Aspirin-containing products can prolong bleeding.
- Tylenol can be substituted for relief of discomfort.

Table 3   Facts needed to interpret and compare results

Laser information
Time course
  Evaluation
  Healing
Age of patient
Color of skin
Location of lesion
Color of lesion
Surface characteristics
Type of anesthesia
Histologic data
Scars
  Hypertrophic
  Atrophic
Pigmentary changes

cosmetic. The *texture of the skin* is often improved, becoming smoother in nature. Gilchrest *et al.*, recently treated a number of patients after having applied ice to the face, and noted marked improvement in the texture [8]. This is understandable in view of the relative nonspecificity of the argon laser and the fact that it does affect the epidermis. By lightening and *breaking up the PWS*, the effect of a solid color 'mass' is either minimized or negated. In certain parts of the face, *the actual size of the lesion treated decreases* from partial disappearance of the lesion, accompanied by a slight contraction of the skin. *Bleeding* is less of a problem after treatment, given the decreased amount of blood flowing through the skin. As noted above, the normal PWS in a number of patients will become progressively ectatic with time, with an associated darkening of the color. This *evolution is stopped* by treatment with the laser beam. In addition, in a number of patients there is a *large psychological* benefit [11].

It is very difficult to assess results of laser treatment to date. Many of the reports have been very small and anecdotal in nature, the results have been interpreted by the same person (people) who performed the treatment, and there have been inadequate or no controls. Some of the reports have been more 'commercial' than scientific in their orientation. There have been few truly scientific studies performed to date. This inadequate assessment is quite understandable given the 'newness' of lasers as a modality of therapy for lesions of the skin. However, in order to interpret and compare the results of both past and future studies, much more information must be provided about the laser, as well as the patients being investigated (see Table 3 and Chapter 2) [24].

The outcome of most studies has shown that a desirable result, defined by marked lightening without scarring, is noted in between 70 and 85 percent of the patients treated. When results are presented they should be broken down by age of patient, color of lesion, color of patient, location of lesion, and histologic parameters. A number of the major studies to date have shown a much higher incidence of scarring when children are included in the evaluation, compared to the results with adults only. Younger patients tend to have poorer results because of the increased incidence of scarring as well as the decreased absolute amount of lightening. Darker lesions tend to respond better then lighter lesions, both in degree of lightening and in flattening of associated hypertrophy. When biopsies are obtained it is clear that the greater the number of red blood cells present in superficial vessels, the more desirable the results. Facial PWS respond better than do PWS on other parts of the body. A greater degree of lightening and a much smaller incidence of scarring are manifested when treatment is on the face.

References

1. Pratt, A. G. Birthmarks in infants. *Arch. Dermatol. Syphilol.* 1953; **67**:302–5.
2. Jacobs, A. H., Walton, R. D. The incidence of birthmarks in the neonate. *Pediatrics.* 1976; **58**:218–22.
3. Barsky, S. H., Rosen, S., Geer, D. E., *et al.* The nature and evolution of port wine stains: a computer-assisted study. *J. Invest. Dermatol.* 1980; **74**:154–7.
4. Glover, J. L., Bendick, P. J., Link, W. J. (Eds). The use of thermal knives in surgery: electrosurgery, lasers, plasma scalpel. *Curr. Probl. Surg.* 1978; **15**:1–78.
5. Fuller, T. A. The physics of lasers. *Lasers in Surgery and Medicine.* 1980; **1**:5–14.
6. Zinn, K. M. Clinical aspects of ophthalmic argon lasers. *Lasers in Surgery and Medicine.* 1981; **1**:289–322.
7. Van Gemert, M. J. C., Hulsbergen-Henning, J. P. A model approach to laser coagulation of dermal vascular lesions. *Arch. Dermatol. Res.* 1981; **270**, 429–439.
8. Gilchrest, B. A., Rosen, S., Noe, J. M. Chilling port wine stains improves the response to argon laser therapy. *Plast. Reconstr. Surg.* 1982; **69**:278–83.
9. Greenwald, J., Rosen, S., Anderson, R. R., *et al.* Comparative histological studies of the tunable dye (at 577 nm) laser and argon laser: the specific vascular effects of the dye laser. *J. Invest. Dermatol.* 1981; **77**:305–10.
10. Noe, J. M., Barsky, S. H., Geer, D. E., *et al.* Port wine stains and the response to argon laser therapy: successful treatment and the predictive role of color, age and biopsy. *Plast. Reconstr. Surg.* 1980; **65**:130–6.
11. Kalick, M., Goldwyn, R. M., Noe, J. M. Social issues and body image concerns of port wine stain patients undergoing laser therapy. *Lasers in Surgery and Medicine.* 1981; **1**:205–13.
12. Finley, J., Barsky, S., Geer, D., *et al.* Healing of port wine stains after argon laser therapy. *Arch. Dermatol.* 1981; **117**:486–9.
13. Apfelberg, D., Kosek, J., Maser, M., *et al.* Histopathology of port wine stains following argon laser tretment. *Br. J. Plast. Surg.* 1979; **32**: 232–7.
14. Solomon, H., Goldman, L., Henderson, B., *et al.* Histopathology of the laser treatment of port wine lesions. *J. Invest. Dermatol.* 1969; **50**:141–6.
15. Ohmori, S. Effect of argon laser beam upon port wine stain (abstr). *ASPRS/ASMS Plastic Surgery Forum.* 1978; **1**:56.
16. Larrow, L., Noe, J. Care of the patient with a port wine stain hemangioma. *Am. J. Nurs.* 1982; **82**:786–90.
17. Arndt, K. A., Burton K., Noe, J. M. Minimizing the pain of local anesthesia. *Plast. Reconstr. Surg.* In press.

18. Apfelberg, D. B., Maser, M. R., Lash, H. Argon laser management of cutaneous vascular deformities: a preliminary report. *West. J. Med.* 1976; **124**: 99–101.
19. Goldman, L. Effects of new laser systems on the skin. *Arch. Dermatol.* 1973; **108**:385–90.
20. Cosman, B. Experience in the argon laser therapy of port wine stains. *Plast. Reconstr. Surg.* 1980; **65**:119–29.
21. Hobby, W. Treatment of port wine stains and other cutaneous lesions. *Contemp. Surg.* 1981; **18**:21–8.
22. Goldman, L., Dreffer, R., Rockwell, J. R., Jr., *et al.* Treatment of port wine marks by an argon laser. *J. Dermatol. Surg.* 1976; **2**:385–8.
23. Goldman, L., Dreffer, R., Laser treatment of extensive mixed cavernous and port-wine stains. *Arch. Dermatol.* 1977; **113**:504–5.
24. Arndt, K. A., Noe, J. M., Northam, D. B. C., *et al.* Laser therapy. Basic concepts and nomenclature. *J. Am. Acad. Dermatol.* 1981; **5**:649–54.

Cutaneous Laser Therapy: Principles and Methods
Edited by K. A. Arndt, J. M. Noe, and S. Rosen
© 1983 John Wiley & Sons Ltd

11

Argon Laser Treatment of Port Wine Stains

John A. Dixon

The appearance of a typical pink/purple port wine stain (PWS) on the face or body of a newborn initiates a traumatic series of events for a patient and parents. The usual reaction of the parents is one of guilt and a feeling that some type of stigma has been attached to the child. Indeed, the word 'stigma' originally was used to describe a mark, burn, or cut that the ancient Greeks used to place upon the body of a moral outcast. The Old Testament talks about the 'Mark of Cain' which was a sign God placed upon a sinner's body so that the world would instantly recognize the sinner. Parents sometimes are reassured by well-meaning but ill-informed health personnel that the lesion is a bruise or a forceps mark or is related to some circumstance of the delivery and will certainly disappear. Confusion frequently exists between the nevus flammeus or PWS which tends to remain through life and the strawberry hemangioma of infancy which in 70 percent of patients disappears by the age of approximately 7 years [1]. The existence of the PWS lesion motivates the parents and later the patient to seek help for this distressing problem. The urgency of concealment of the lesion is illustrated by one mother in our series who went to a newborn nursery early every morning and applied cover makeup to the PWS on the face of an infant daughter. The other age extreme is illustrated by a patient who had been married 32 years and insisted her husband was not aware of the lesion inasmuch as she would arise an hour or two before her husband and laboriously apply cover makeup every day.

It is difficult to determine the exact incidence of PWS inasmuch as such concealment does not lend itself to accurate reporting. It appears in approximately one in every 300 live births [2]. Although lesions may occur in kindreds, the lesion does not appear to be genetically related [3].

Syndromes associated with the appearance of the PWS include Sturge–Weber, in which PWS is present in approximately 5 percent of patients [2], and Klippel–Trenaunay (see Chapter 8). The interesting distribution of PWS of the face seems related to the trigeminal nerve with the lesion occupying the skin area of V_1, V_2, V_3, or any combination of these. Of further interest is the observation by Stevenson and Morin [4] that in patients with involvement of V_1 and V_2 by PWS, there is a 15 percent chance of glaucoma being present and a 30 percent chance of glaucoma ultimately developing (see Chapter 9).

The great majority of lesions appear on the face, followed by the trunk, the neck, the lower and upper extremities [5]. The lesions initially are light pink and flat. It is interesting that in 3 percent of patients in this series, the mother did not notice the discoloration until 3–6 hours following birth, after which it became progressively more evident. Following puberty, the lesions appear to darken, going from pink to deep red or purple. In patients past 30 years of age, 50–60 percent of facial lesions will begin to undergo a nodular, 'bubly', or cavernous change [2]. The lesions will protrude 2–3 mm and tend to sag. The protrusions over the eyelid and mouth are discomforting and disfiguring. The etiology of this change is unknown but is thought to be a degeneration of the supportive structures of the skin. It is also speculated that the progressive ectasia of the vessels due to shunting of blood may produce this change.

Because of the distressing nature of the PWS, numerous therapies have been tried. Excision and skin graft has been one of the methods most frequently employed. This has had all the disadvantages of multiple procedures, scarring of donor sites, inadequate and inappropriate match of donor skin to adjacent facial skin, and scarring. Tattooing with flesh-colored pigments has likewise been undertaken. This is less than satisfactory due to the problems of matching of color plus a tendency of the tattooed area to lighten as the pigment tends to migrate, as well as lightening due to a process of phagocytosis [6]. Additional modalities of treatment have included x-ray and cryotherapy with dry ice. These have provided only temporary relief and significant scarring in some cases.

The use of the argon laser with a wavelength in the 488- to 518-nm bands was reported favorably by Apfelberg *et al.*, in 1976 [7]. Since that time a number of additional reports of good results have appeared [2,3,5,8–10]. The argon laser was suggested because of the selective absorption of blue-green light by the red-purple hemoglobin chromagen of the PWS [11]. In-as-much as it is necessary to discuss possible outcomes of treatment in the pretreatment interview with a patient being considered for argon laser therapy of PWS, the results of our series and those of other reported series will be discussed here rather than at the conclusion of the chapter as is customary in presentations of this type. This information is essential in preoperative discussions with the patient concerning the potential benefits and hazards relating to the procedures they are possibly going to undergo.

Results of treatment

The University of Utah series consisted of 73 patients followed for more than 1 year after argon therapy for PWS. Of this group, 13 were under 12 years of age, 60 were over 12 years of age. Because of marked differences of outcomes of treatments which will be discussed later, the results of those under and over 12 will be discussed separately. There were 40 females and 33 males in the overall series with a mean age of 24.8 years and an age range from 9 to 83 years. The mean number of treatments per patient was 2.6, including many small 'touch-up' treatments. The classification of results is that proposed by Apfelberg *et al*, with categories of *excellent* (total blanching without scar), *good* (marked lightening without scar), *poor* (no change), and *scar* [9]. Of the group of 60 treated patients over 12 years of age, 8.6 percent were classified as excellent, 81.1 percent as good, 6.9 percent as poor, and 3.4 percent had significant scarring. Illustrations of excellent and good results are seen in Figures 1, 2, and 3. Significant scarring in a young patient is seen in Figure 4. In the group of 13 patients under 12 years of age, 7.6 percent had an excellent result, 50.8 percent good results, 26.6 percent poor results, and 15 percent had significant scarring.

Because of the difference in age groups and reporting categories, it is difficult to tabulate in parallel the various series discussed in this chapter. This is attempted in Table 1. It should be noted that the age groups are not all the same in each series and the categories do not read consistently across headings. The comparison is made in the form reported by each author so as not to do violence to their intent.

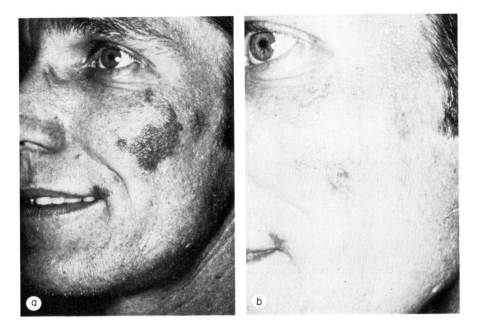

Figure 1   Port wine stain. (*a*) Pretreatment appearance. (*b*) Excellent result.
Complete removal of color. No scarring or pigmentation

The comparison does allow certain generalities. It appears that in only
approximately 8 percent of patients will the PWS be completely removed.
Approximately 70 percent of treated patients will obtain a good to fair result
with variable degrees of lightening, 15 percent will show little or no change, and
5–7 percent will have significant scarring.

These results suggest that, as recommended by Kalick and his associates
[12] (and see Chapter 20), a proper presentation of outcomes to the
patient would emphasize 'lightening' rather than 'removal' of the PWS
inasmuch as the great majority of patients do indeed have remaining PWS
following treatment.

The treated patient's perception of these results as identified in the Utah
series will be discussed later in this chapter. It should be emphasized that in a
procedure of this type the true outcome is that which is perceived by the patient
rather than by over- or underoptimistic numbers of the treatment team.
Experience with a group of over 200 patients with PWS suggests that a
carefully organized realistic approach to the patient, his/her lesion, and laser
therapy will produce the most beneficial results and greatest patient
satisfaction. The steps in such treatment are outlined for convenience in Table
2 and are further discussed under subsequent headings.

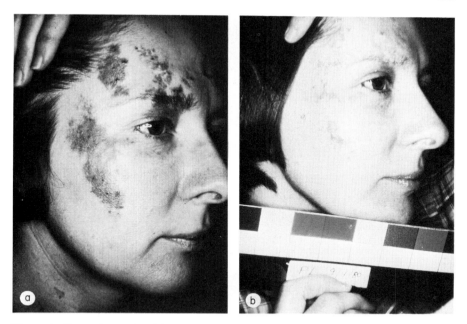

Figure 2   Port wine stain. (*a*) Pretreatment appearance. (*b*) Good result. No scarring. Lesion much lighter. Some residual deep vessel pattern

Pretreatment interview

One of the most important procedures in the entire therapeutic process is the pretreatment interview with the patient and family. This interview may be conducted by any one or all of the laser treatment team which may consist of a physician, nurse practitioner, and psychologist. It is essential at this time to elicit a careful history to determine the family's and the patient's attitudes toward the lesion and the expectations of each relative to the therapeutic process. The natural history of the disease is discussed and many previous notions relative to the disease confirmed or eliminated. It is essential to know who is bothered most by the PWS—the patient, the mother, the father, or other associates. Patients submitting grudgingly to treatment as a result of outside pressures frequently are difficult to guide through a course of therapy and much less appreciative of results. The entire lasery therapy treatment is discussed in detail with the patient, with particular emphasis on the appearance of the lesion in the immediate postoperative period including weeping, discharge, crusting, the possibility of no change or scarring, and probabilities of lightening. It is particularly important to stress that it may require as long as 1–2 years before the ultimate result will be obtained and that the immediate

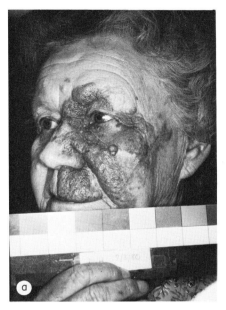

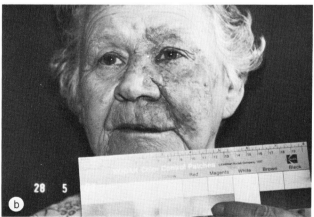

Figure 3   Port wine stain. (*a*) Hypertrophic, bubbly PWS pretreatment. (*b*) Good
result. Marked flattening. Good color change

result of therapy may be a lighter pink color as healing takes place, which only
later will be replaced by the desired blanching. It should be noted that many
times the lesion will blanch unevenly following treatment and that mild degrees
of hyper- or hypopigmentation may be present. The mottling and pigmentation
will usually improve in 6–12 months. It is useful to have a book of pre- and
post-therapy photographs of other patients illustrating excellent, good, fair,

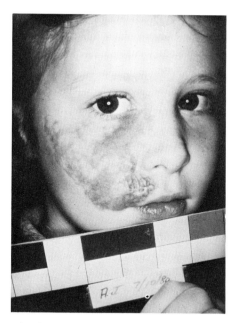

Figure 4   Port wine stain. Scarring in upper lip of 9-year-old. General improvement
of color

poor results, and scarring for all to see. As the study by Kalick *et al.* [12]
indicates, despite the most careful explanation of projected outcomes and
possible hazards, a high percentage of individuals will deny that the possibility
of scarring was ever discussed with them. The review of pictures serves to
further impress the patient with these possibilities and makes for reasonable
expectations.

It is important to question the patient carefully regarding scarring from
previous operations, injuries, or even vaccinations. A tendency to keloid
formation (and hence, a contraindication to laser therapy) may be identified by
this inquiry.

At this point it is usually possible to describe in a general way to the patient
the statistical probabilities of the various aspects of treatment benefits,
hazards, and risks involved. As with any surgical procedure, the patient and
family will want to know the probabilities of benefits to be expected and costs
and risks encountered. Utilizing the results of our series and others previously
described, it is now possible to list and quantitate in a general way the answers
to these questions. For convenient reference, the benefits and hazards with
approximate figures for each are shown in Table 3 and Table 4. An
amplification on some of these factors follows.

Table 1 Collected results of argon laser therapy of port wine stains

	No. of patients	Results				
		Excellent	Good	Fair	Poor	Scar
Apfelberg et al.	130	11	68		34	17
Cosman	33	1	18	12	2	2
Dixon						
> 12 years of age	60	8.6%	81.1%		6.9%	3.4%
< 12 years of age	13	7.6%	50.8%		26.6%	15%
Noe et al.	62	Desirable: 73%	Undesirable: 27%	Scar: 11%		

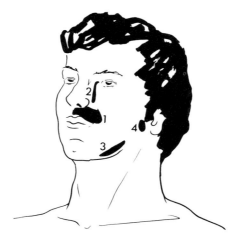

Figure 5   Severity of scarring (PWS, argon laser). Number 1 indicates site of most
frequent and severe scarring; other sites in decreasing order

Table 2   Port wine stains: treatment steps

Pretreatment interview
Selection factors
Informed consent
Photography
Selection of anesthesia
Treatment
Postoperative follow-up
Management of scarring

Table 3   Port wine stains: treatment benefits

Decrease or eliminate abnormal color	85%
Break up solid color mass	7%
Texture/elevation improvement (? arrest)	95%
Elimination of bleeding	90%

In the treatment benefit category, it has been noted that, in addition to
decreasing overall color of the lesions, laser therapy will frequently result in
irregular areas of lightening which tend to break up the visual impression of
solid colored mass. Some of the far-advanced lesions in older patients present a
nodular or bubbly texture and are elevated. Flattening of these lesions
frequently is beneficial. At this time it is not known whether laser therapy

Table 4   Port wine stains: hazards of treatment

Hypertrophic scarring	6%
Hyper/hypopigmentation	7%
Infection, invasive	2%
Pain—minimal to moderate	90%
Anesthetic risk	1:10,000
Time	2–3 weeks
Ocular injury	0
Cost—professional, laser, hospital	Individual

prevents the progression of the juvenile lesion to carvernous transformation and elevation. Four percent of patients had a history of rupture of one or more cavernous areas of the lesion with bleeding. Such bleeding is usually eliminated with therapy.

On the hazards or cost side of the ledger, scarring is the most disconcerting occurrence and should be discussed openly with the patient. The hyper- or hypopigmentation usually resolves in 8–12 months. This is particularly a problem in Caucasians with darker skin. Treatment in non-Caucasians is more difficult in that a whitish area of hypopigmentation is very poorly tolerated. Reported experiences with laser treatment are minimal in the races with heavily pigmented skin in this country, although a large series has been reported in Japan with good results (S. Ohmori, personal communication). Pain is surprisingly minimal and is considerably less than would be noted with thermal burns of equal extent. Anesthetic risks should be mentioned as general anesthesia has a morbidity of 4 per 10,000 and local anesthetic a lesser figure [13]. With extensive treated lesions of the face, it is difficult for the patient to continue to work because of unpleasant appearance; time lost from work may be from 2 to 5 weeks. To all of this must be added the financial cost of the treatment which varies greatly with the extent of the lesion, treatment setting, anesthetic used (local or general), and number of treatments required.

Selection factors

Having discussed the general probabilities of various outcomes with the patient, a number of selection factors can then be employed in order to increase the likelihood of a good result and reduce the possibilities of no improvement or scarring. These factors are listed in Table 5 and a detailed discussion follows.

There is now general agreement that children do less well than adults. The exact 'cut off' age varies in various series from 12 to 15 years [3,6]. It is interesting that the Japanese experience as described by Ohmori includes children of all ages with reported good results. There is general correlation of the biopsies in the younger age groups with small, underfilled, straight vessels and pink color [6].

Table 5   Port wine stains: selection factors

Age	Over 15
Location	Face, neck
Biopsy	Less than 1 mm, plump vessels
Test patches	No scar, good color change
Color coding	Deeper reds, purple
Blanching	Minimal
Blood velocity and flow	Not fully evaluated

Lesions on the face seem to do better than those on the neck. Lesions of both extremities, trunk, and especialy anterior chest, have lesser reduction in color and a higher incidence of scarring.

The elegant study of Noe *et al.* [6] has shown that lesions that are less than 1 mm in depth with ectatic superficial vessels with a high percentage of filling with red blood cells respond better to argon laser therapy than vessels of smaller diameter with less filling or deeper placement in the lesions.

The treatment of a small area of the lesion—a 'test patch'—has been a useful method of selection. There is approximately a 60 percent correlation of test patch results wherein no scar and good color change in the test area predict a good eventual outcome [3]. There is, however, a considerable number of cases of patients with poor test patches who do much better than predicted and others with good test patches but with poor results. This probably relates to nonhomogeneity of the lesions.

Color coding of the PWS using various types of standards has been employed. Noe *et al.* [6] found that color generally correlated with the more superficial, plumper vessels and with biopsy. The deeper reds and purples in all series have a higher percentage of favorable results than do the light pink and red hues. Spectrophotometric studies (see Chapter 3) are in process at our institution. The attempt is to more definitively predict the pattern of reflectance and absorption that will respond most favorably to the argon laser based upon a determination of the complete spectrum of absorption and reflectance of a given lesion. The work is preliminary at this time.

Cosman [3] has suggested that blanching on pressure is a poor prognostic sign. The etiologic reasons for this are not evident at this time. It is postulated that the nonblanchers may have a more static blood flow which is more amenable to laser therapy.

Studies are under way at our institution using the Halloway helium neon laser Doppler velocimeter in an effort to map blood flow in the PWS to determine the relationships of the dynamics of blood flow to outcome of laser therapy [14]. At the present time the results are interesting but not sufficiently far advanced to provide predictive information.

Informed consent

Despite widespread application of the argon laser for PWS, it is essential to provide the patient with all possible information so that they can make an informed decision relative to their treatment. Some institutions require special forms indicating that the procedure is of a research nature and requires approval of an Institutional Review Committee. In a community hospital situation, it would be well for the therapist to develop, in cooperation with a lawyer, an appropriate consent form for their setting.

Photographs

Photographs are taken of all lesions pre- and postoperatively. A Kodak color bar is included so as to provide a color reference and allow evaluation of differences in exposure. These photographs are essential in later evaluation of results for direction of therapy or counselling of patients. Signed permission for use of such photographs is necessary if they are to be used in scientific publications.

Anesthesia

Inasmuch as anesthesia is required to a depth of only 1 mm, our group undertook extensive studies with regard to relatively noninvasive types of local anesthesia, including topical anesthetic pastes applied to the skin with occlusive dressings, iontophoresis, regional nerve block, and the use of penetrants such as DMSO (dimethylsulfoxide). None of these provides satisfactory anesthesia except DMSO plus lidocaine. In this situation, however, the DMSO produced such local erythema of the skin as to make the correct color tones and margins of normal skin and PWS almost impossible to detect. Regional nerve blocks are helpful but frequently more uncomfortable than regional infiltration. Current practice is to use either intradermal infiltration with a local anesthetic or general anesthesia. Local anesthesia is elected when the lesions are relatively small and confluent and the patient is adult and stable. Lesions that have multiple noncontiguous stains are less well treated by this method. Light general anesthesia is employed in apprehensive patients, patients with large lesions that would require more than the maximum permissive dose of local anesthesia, and patients with nonconfluent lesions. General anesthesia multiplies the costs to the patient several times, however.

Procedure

The laser equipment employed for the treatment of PWS is usually an argon laser transmitting several lines between 488 and 512 nm. A flexible quartz waveguide of 400-μm or 600-μm diameter is used to transmit energy from the power source to the area of treatment. Some small metallic terminal device is usually provided for ease in holding the fiber tip. The beam projected is usually concentric with a Gaussian distribution of the irradiance across the treated area. A device projecting a rectangular spot for special usage has been developed by D. W. Auth (personal communication).

Other chapters in this volume have described the method of determination of energy density or, more properly, irradiance per cm^2. In general (see Chapter 2), there are two methods of applying the argon laser—intermittent and continuous. In the intermittent technique a time setting such as 0.2 sec and a spot size of 2 mm are selected. The power setting is adjusted to 0.6–0.8 W. One spot application is then made to the anesthetized skin. The resulting desired spot should be clear and distinct with good blanching of the vessels. The overlying epidermis should be white with no initial gray or black coloration. The power is gradually adjusted upward from the 0.6–0.8 W level with successive spots until this end is achieved. At the point when this level is determined (usually between 0.8 and 1.4 W) an interval between spot applications is then selected. This usually results in a formula such as 1 W delivered for a duration of 0.2 sec with an interval of 0.5–1 sec. At a fixed distance, the calculated irradiance from such a treatment formula is 30 J/cm^2. When using the continuous technique, the power setting is initially determined exactly as for the intermittent technique using a 0.2-sec application. Once the power level has been adjusted, the laser source is switched from intermittent to continuous application and the speed of transit of the fiber across the skin determined by blanching of the PWS. The variable speed of transit results in varying power densities, generally approximating 20–40 J/cm^2. Variations in blanching may be noted in various areas of a given PWS. If, when using the intermittent technique, the spot appears to become larger, more absorption is taking place and the power should be reduced. Reduction in spot size indicates lesser absorption and the need for higher power levels. The same thing may be noted in the continuous technique by narrowing or widening of the continuous line. Moving the fiber more slowly or more rapidly across the skin will produce the same effect as altering the power level. In practice, either adjustment may be made with satisfactory results.

Application

With the lesion anesthetized and the source power level and irradiance determined, actual application begins. In the intermittent technique, spots are applied in a linear fashion such that the margins of the blanching intersect but do not overlap. In the continuous technique, the fiber is held approximately 1–3 cm from the skin (depending upon the angle of divergence of the beam used) and passed across the skin as rapidly as necessary to provide blanching of the PWS. If the epidermis is white and the vessels have blanched, an appropriate irradiance has been applied. Minimal change in the epidermis without blanching usually means inadequate power density and inadequate irradiance. Blanching with dark gray to black skin or blistering means excessive irradiance and appropriate correction should be made.

There are two general patterns of PWS photocoagulation. In one, stripping or spotting is utilized, leaving alternate 2–3 mm wide bands untreated. Alternate lines are treated at a later sitting. In the confluent technique, the entire lesion is photocoagulated with each line of application abutting but not overlapping the next. It has been our practice to use the confluent technique except over the eyelids, the upper lip, and the upper portion of the lower lip. Inasmuch as the vascular bed is altered by the initial striping treatment and healing, it has been difficult to match exactly the color and stripe margins at subsequent applications months later.

In the case of the ligher-colored lesions, it is useful to outline the PWS with a skin marker as the margins sometimes appear less distinct as the therapy proceeds. It is best to complete one area of the lesion completely rather than move to another area and return, as a histamine flare appears in treated areas after 2–3 minutes which creates a temporary erythema that is difficult to distinguish from the remaining PWS. One can then get caught in a cycle of retreating a treated area where a reaction to injury looks like untreated PWS.

Eye protection

When lesions are outside the areas of the eye, protective goggles such as Laser Gard are worn by the patient. For lesions involving the malar, zygomatic, periorbital, and brow regions it is usually sufficient to tape a moist sponge on the contralateral eye and for the operator to hold a sponge firmly over the eye on the involved side. The patient should be cautioned to report seeing any blue-green light. This protection is satisfactory for all lesions except those involving the lids themselves. Methods vary for treatment of lesions of the lids. Our method is to anesthetize the cornea and conjunctiva with Ophthaine drops, elevate the lids with lid retractors, and insert a lead contact shield such as is used by radiotherapists. When the treatment is completed, the shield is removed immediately to avoid the possibility of corneal injury. Shields of less bulky material are also available. Some individuals feel that heavy infiltration of local anesthetic thickening the subcutaneous tissue is sufficient barrier to passage of the argon laser without inserting any type of eye shield. While this may be true, the insertion of positive eye protection reassures the apprehensive patient and provides better legal protection for the operator from subsequent litigation should the patient develop any unrelated ocular difficulty at a later date. Protective goggles are worn by the operator and by all individuals in the room while laser is operational or therapy is in progress.

Treatment of lips

While the upper lip should be striped or spotted, the vermilion border should be treated as a continuous line. Spotting or striping that crosses the vermilion border results in a notched appearance which is undesirable and difficult to avoid. Our practice is to delineate the vermilion border with one precise continuous linear application, then spot the upper lip in an irregular reticular pattern with very careful attention to power settings and blanching as previously described.

Treatment of external ear

Questions frequently arise relative to treatment of the external ear. Just as with the upper lip, the ear lobe appears to be somewhat more sensitive, although scarring has not been encountered in this area. Because of the underlying ear cartilage we have treated only one side of the external ear at one sitting. Irradiance along the margin of the ear is carefully controlled. Injury of the cartilage has not been encountered, but experience with thermal burns suggests care in this area. The eyebrows and eyelids are not shaved. With care, the hairs may be retracted from one side to the other and short applications of the laser applied around the hair follicles. It has not been found necessary to remove all PWS in the brows. If the solid color mass is broken up and the areas between the hairs of the brow lightened, a very acceptable cosmetic result is obtained even though the entire lesion has not been obliterated.

Effect of post-treatment cooling

Considerable diversity of opinion exists relative to cooling immediately following the laser treatment of PWS. It is felt that such cooling may reduce the heating of the normal tissue and dermis and reduce the incidence of scarring [9]. Other studies suggest that such cooling might creat ischemia, especially on large lesions, and result in deeper penetration [15]. It is our practice at this time to use cooling by ice or disposable cold chemical bags only when treatment is conducted around the eyes where considerable postoperative swelling takes place.

Postoperative care

The general aim of postoperative care is to keep the wound clean, dry, and as free as possible from foreign substances and infection. Lesions are bandaged only where clothes are likely to rub and produce irritation. A thin film of bacitracin ointment is applied. The patient is instructed regarding the appearance of some vesiculation, drainage, and encrustation. Although showering is allowed, the patient is requested not to pull at the crust but to allow it to separate spontaneously. A thin film of ointment is used until the crusts have separated. Care is used not to apply excessive ointment and produce maceration of the treated area. After the crusts have separated, the previously stained area frequently will be a light pink due to the erythema of healing such as seen following a thermal burn. The patient is informed of this appearance and reassured that blanching will occur over a period of 6–12 weeks. Due to the unpredictable reaction of the laser-treated melanocytes, patients are requested to wear a sunscreen with a sun protection factor of 15 or higher over the treated area whenever they are exposed to sunlight, for a period of approximately 1 year. The treated area tends to react to sunlight by irregular pigmentation or even undesirable freckling. For convenience, a postoperative care sheet is utilized by our clinic similar to that given in Table 2 of Chapter 10. With regard to the care of the lips, lower neck, and ears, because of the increased incidence of scarring, Valisone ointment 0.1 percent is recommended.

The frequency of postoperative visits is quite variable depending upon the size of the lesion, geographic distance from physician, etc. It was with some reluctance that we initially treated 10–12 square inches of the face and then allowed the patient to travel some thousands of miles distant from the clinic. As a practical matter, the only circumstances requiring early postoperative attention are invasive infection and scarring. When starting this type of therapy, the operator may wish to see the patient every 3–4 days or weekly, then every month for 3 months. Ultimately, however, most patients will be instructed to return in 3 months unless infection or scarring supervenes. If proper instruction is given pre- and postoperatively to the patient with regard to identification of these complications and the need to report them immediately to the clinic, untoward results and frequent troublesome visits may be avoided. In general, where patients do not have to travel too far, they are seen in 3 months and again in 1 year. No retreatments are undertaken until at least 1 year has elapsed. We have noted lightening of lesions continuing as long as 18 months.

Retreatment

Fifteen patients have undergone retreatment of an entire lesion that failed to lighten. Of these 15, six noted further overall lightening of their lesion; eight were unimproved. No additional tendency toward scarring was noted. Many of our patients have required 'touch-up' of small areas that were missed or looked darker than other portions of the treated lesion. These generally respond very favorably. It is our feeling at this time that additional treatment is useful for missed areas or areas where discrete patches of vessels that seemed to be somewhat deeper than the overall lesion are still evident. Treatment of an entire lesion when the overall improvement has been less than satisfactory has been rewarding in less than 50 percent of our patients.

Discussion

Frequent reference has been made here to the complication of scarring. It is certainly most distressing to the patient and to the physician to make an already unsightly lesion worse. Scarring, therefore, becomes the major complication and hazard in argon laser therapy of PWS. The overall incidence of scarring has been listed in Table 1. Further comment concerning this distressing problem is indicated, however. Although selective absorption by the chromagen hemoglobin in vessels certainly does take place, it is evident both experimentally and clinically that sufficient absorption of the epidermis and upper layers of the dermis does occur to produce thermal injury extending into the papillary dermis [16,17]. If this is the case, the patient then becomes hostage to scarring, just as any patient with a thermal burn, with the outcome dependent upon a multiplicity of factors such as the healing tendencies of the patient, the presence of superficial or deep infection, the occurrence of trauma to the healing wound (such as avulsion of crusts), the presence of motion or traction upon the healing lesion, and the intrusion of foreign bodies (dust, cosmetic, etc.) into the healing lesion. Thus it might be said, using a strict histologic definition of increased collagen and fibrous deposition in the skin, that all patients treated with argon laser have scarring, just as all patients following a surgical incision have scarring. What is important, then, is objectionable scarring or scarring that is more prominent than the initial vascular lesion. R. H. Rotering (personal communication) has made a study of the patient's perception of the area of his/her PWS following laser therapy. It is interesting that 86 percent of patients reported that they had some 'scarring'. Further investigation revealed that 'scarring' referred to by the patient consisted of any aspect of the treated area that had a less satisfactory appearance than the patient expected. Close questioning revealed that patients defined scarring as any area that was elevated or indented, darker or lighter in color, rougher or smoother, or in any way noticeable. In only 6 percent of such patients, however, was this recognizable area ultimately considered to be true scarring and objectionable. It is entirely possible that the extensive prelaser therapy discussion of the possible side effects of this modality, including scarring, resulted in some of these patients' identification. It is important, therefore, to define what is meant by scarring when recording results. The Utah group used a scale based on height, color, and extent of the lesion. Based on this scale, the team felt that 3.4 percent of patients with PWS over age 12 had objectionable scarring of grade 3 or greater (over 5 mm extent, greater than 1 mm elevation, color red or darker). In patients under the age of 12, 15 percent had scarring of grade 3 or greater. Gradual improvement has been noted in all patients with scarring. To date none has required surgical correction.

Prevention is certainly the most important solution to the problem of scarring. Selection factors as previously described are most important. The exclusion of the patient with a tendency toward keloid formation or with a test patch demonstrating excess of fibrous reaction will reduce the incidence of this problem. In our observation, by all odds the most important predictive factor is age. As previously mentioned, in our series there was a five times greater incidence of scarring under the age of 12 than in patients over the age of 12. The reasons for this are unknown at this time, but probably relate to the very thin epidermis and dermis of young people combined with smaller, less ectatic vessels requiring higher energy densities for blanching. The anatomic location of the lesion is likewise of great important. This is represented diagnostically in Figure 5 with the upper lip being the site of the most frequent and severe scarring, followed by the nasolabial fold, medial canthus of the eye, mandibular and preauricular areas. Scarring may be reduced in these areas by careful attention to power densities, using the minimal amount to produce blanching, and by resorting to a spotting, reticular, or striping pattern with treatment provided in a two-stage fashion. Appropriate postoperative wound care to avoid infection and trauma is likewise useful.

Scarring has been noted as early as 3 weeks or as late as 3 months following laser treatment. It is interesting that patients will usually say that there has been some discomfort and tightness in the area. Some report a stinging sensation. Following this, there is the appearance of a firm nodule which then progressively enlarges. Patients are instructed to report immediately any unusual stinging or discomfort appearing in a healing lesion later than 3 weeks following treatment.

Inasmuch as nearly 85 percent of patients will have some residual of the PWS or the treatment, it has proved useful to have the assistance of a cosmetologist. Many patients already have some experience in the use of various covering agents, but this is frequently fragmentary and cost ineffective. The cosmetologist consults with the patient during or at the completion of treatment. An individualized program that is most beneficial and least expensive is suggested, depending upon the patient's needs. It is worthy of note that, prior to treatment, some patients spend as much as $400 to $500 per year on covering agents.

Once identified, a variety of treatments have been employed to reduce scarring. Intralesional steroid injections (triamcinolone acetonide, 40 mg/ml) has appeared to reduce the inflammatory response. Lesser lesions are treated by the application of steroid-impregnated tape (flurandrenolone tape) which may be cut in a pattern of the scar and applied to the lesion with tape changes every 12 hours. Smaller, less prominent scars are treated by corticosteroid cream massaged into the lesion four times a day. Scars of the hand, wrist, ankle, etc. are greatly improved by the application of a Jobst pressure support which is kept on at all times except for bathing, etc. Experience in our Burn Unit would indicate these pressure supports would be useful on the face. They must, however, be worn almost constantly for a period of 9–12 months to be effective. Continuous wearing of a mask-like support is not tolerated by most people.

Conclusions

In summary, the argon laser appears to be a very useful modality in the treatment of PWS. It is very important for the physician to discuss thoroughly the nature of the lesion with the patient and family, including the probable progression as age advances. Results from application of the laser should be couched in terms of 'lightened' rather than 'removed'. The treatment is rapid and relatively painless. The major complication is scarring, which can be dramatically reduced by the application of selection factors such as age and by special care in scar-prone areas. At various centers efforts are being directed toward a noninvasive colorimetric, spectrophotometric, or blood flow selection method that would identify and eliminate those patients who would likely have minimal to no lightening of their lesion with treatment. It is hoped that investigations such as those being conducted by Anderson and Parrish with regard to more selective laser wavelengths that would increase vascular injury and concomitantly reduce injury to the skin will assist further with the scarring problem [11] (and see Chapter 4). At this time, however, it is unclear whether or not the cosmetic result judged as desirable by the patient may be to some degree determined by the whitening produced by the scarring of the epidermis and dermis in addition to the obliteration of the vessels.

Distressing as it may be to physicist and engineer friends, a final note must be added. Argon laser therapy of PWS is at present an art form. Despite the careful formulations and calculations, the ultimate clinical result depends upon hand–eye coordination of the laser operator to get the color 'just right'. In the intermittent technique, spots must be carefully approximated, stripes carefully matched, and margins blended. In the continuous technique, the point of impact of the laser must be meticulously observed so as to move along at the precise rate necessary. Experienced operators have been observed to employ an almost infinite number of small hand maneuvers such as moving closer or farther from the skin to change irradiance per cm^2, changing beam angle slightly, using edge of spot for slightly less power density, overlapping edges of spots to increase effect, etc. An understanding of physical principles, a visual understanding of laser–skin interactions, and a healthy portion of just plain craftsmanship seem to combine for the best results in argon laser treatment of PWS.

References

1. Bowers, R. E., Graham, E. A., Tomlinson K. M. The natural history of the strawberry nevus. *Arch. Dermatol.* 1960; **82**:59–72.
2. Jacobs, H. A., Walton, R. G. The incidence of birthmarks in the neonate. *Pediatrics.* 1976; **58**:218–22.
3. Cosman, B. Experience in the argon laser therapy of port wine stains. *Plast. Reconstr. Surg.* 1980; **65**:119–29.
4. Stevenson, R. F., Morin, J. D. Ocular findings in nevus flammeus. *Can. J. Ophthalmol.* 1975; **10**:136–40.
5. Hobby, L. W. Treatment of port wine stains and other cutaneous lesions. *Contemp. Surg.* 1981; **18**:22–45.
6. Noe, J. M., Barsky, S. A., Geer, D. E., *et al.* Port wine stains and the response to argon laser therapy: successful treatment and the predictive role of color, age and biopsy. *Plast. Reconstr. Surg.* 1980; **65**:130–5.
7. Apfelberg, D. B., Maser, M. R., Lash, H. Argon laser management of cutaneous vascular deformities. *West. J. Med.* 1976; **124**:99–101.
8. Cosman, B. Argon laser therapy of port wine stains. *J. Med. Soc. NJ.* 1980; **77**:167–74.
9. Apfelberg, D. B., Maser, M. R., Lash, H. Extended clinical use of the argon laser for cutaneous lesions. *Arch. Dermatol.* 1979; **115**:719–21.
10. Apfelberg, D. B., Maser, M. R., Lash, H., *et al.* The argon laser for cutaneous lesions. *JAMA.* 1981; **245**:2073–5.
11. Anderson, R. R., Parrish, J. A. Optical properties of human skin. In: *The Science of Photomedicine.* New York: Plenum Press, 1980; 147–194.
12. Kalick, M. S., Goldwyn, R. M., Noe, J. M. Social issues and body image concerns of port wine stain patients undergoing laser therapy. *Lasers in Surgery and Medicine.* 1981; **1**:205–13.
13. Phillips, J. C. Public health aspects of critical care medicine and anesthesiology. Anesthesia mortality. *Clinical Anesthesia.* 1974; **10**:220.
14. Hollaway, G. A., Watkins, D. W. Laser Doppler measurement of cutaneous blood flow. *J. Invest. Dermatol.* 1977; **69**:306–9.
15. Demling, R. H., Mazess, R. B., Wolberg, W. The effect of immediate and delayed cold immersion on burn edema formation and resorption. *J. Trauma.* 1979; **19**:56–9.
16. Apfelberg, D. B., Kosek, J., Maser, M. R., *et al.* Histology of port wine stains following argon laser treatment. *Br. J. Plast. Surg.* 1979; **32**:232–7.
17. van Gemert, M. J. C., Hulsbergen-Henning, J. P. A model approach to laser coagulation of dermal vascular lesions. *Arch. Dermatol. Res.* 1981; **270**:429–39.

Cutaneous Laser Therapy: Principles and Methods
Edited by K. A. Arndt, J. M. Noe, and S. Rosen
© 1983 John Wiley & Sons Ltd

12

Treatment of Port Wine Stains with the CO_2 laser: Early Results

Philip L. Bailin

Port wine stains (PWS) have presented a major therapeutic challenge to physicians of several disciplines. These lesions are cosmetically disfiguring, often requiring the afflicted patient to spend hours daily in the difficult and tedious procedure of applying opaque makeup. Many patients suffer significant psychosocial impairment as a consequence of their lesions. Furthermore, many patients experience the formation of papulonodular vascular blebs on the surface of the PWS, leading to hemorrhage or surface erosion and secondary infection.

The character of these lesions, including natural history, histology, and earlier forms of therapy, is discussed in other chapters. This chapter will deal with the application of the CO_2 laser to the therapy of PWS.

Several different laser systems have been utilized to treat this condition [1–4]. The argon laser has recently become the preferred modality among most laser surgeons (5–14). This has been covered in Chapters 10 and 11, but an important aspect must be reviewed. The argon laser emits light of two wavelengths, 488 nm and 515 nm. This is in the blue-green portion of the visible spectrum. The *theoretical* basis of argon laser therapy of vascular lesions is that this light energy is more selectively absorbed by the complementary red pigment of blood cells (hemoglobin) than by surrounding cutaneous elements.

However, in practice, such selectivity is not so apparent. Investigators have demonstrated that argon laser light at therapeutic power density levels does indeed damage nonvascular cutaneous structures including epidermis, dermal connective tissue, and adnexal elements. This may be due to heat transmission from the primarily vascular site of absorption, or it may be related to the fact that argon laser light has a relatively high scatter factor in tissue and a high coefficient of extinction in tissue, meaning that the light may travel a considerable distance before being totally absorbed.

Several clinical studies performed with argon lasers have shown that therapy of PWS yielded undesirable results (fair to poor resolution of the lesion) in 23–42 percent of patients [6,8,10,14] and hypertrophic scar formation in 9–23.5 percent (8,10,14). This indicated that there was still room for considerable improvement in the laser therapy of PWS.

Thus, it was decided to treat a group of patients with PWS with the CO_2 laser. The theoretical rationale for such therapy was based upon the characteristics of CO_2 laser light emission.

The active medium of the CO_2 laser is a gas comprised of CO_2, nitrogen, and helium in a ratio of 1:1.5:4. When this medium is pumped via electrical discharge, radiation is generated having a characteristic wavelength of 10,600 nm (far-infrared range). Such radiation is invisible and therefore not *selectively* absorbed by any pigment. It is instead uniformly absorbed in water (or tissue) in a very localized fashion. The scatter is minimal (approximately 7 percent of that of argon laser radiation) and the beam is fully absorbed in only 0.1–0.2 mm of tissue compared to > 4.0 mm of tissue with argon. Moreover, the tissue absorbing the CO_2 laser radiation is instantaneously vaporized at 100 °C. Immediately adjacent tissue is spared and thermal transmission is minimal, extending no more than 30–50 μm from the laser impact site [15]. Thus, the CO_2 laser is far more focal and localized in its tissue-damaging effects than is the argon laser.

Additionally, the CO_2 laser beam seals blood vessels of up to 0.5 mm in diameter on impact. It also has been demonstrated to seal nerve endings [16], which may decrease postoperative discomfort.

The principle, then, in using the CO_2 laser to treat PWS is to vaporize away the cutaneous surface and seal off the vascular network just below the surface. Thermal damage to the remaining tissue bed and peripheral tissue is at a theoretical minimum, allowing for healing with minimal scar formation.

Method of treatment

All patients selected for CO_2 laser therapy have been Caucasian and postpubertal. No patients with documented systemic angiomatosis have been treated. Cosmetic and medical improvement were the goals of therapy. Several patients had previously undergone therapy to portions of their lesions including tattooing with opaque pigments, cryosurgery, and laser therapy (ruby, argon). The eyelid and upper lip areas were excluded prospectively because of the reported higher incidence of scar formation with other therapeutic modalities. Lesions of the trunk and extremities were accepted. Lesions were evaluated as to degree of blanching with pressure, color (pink, red, purple), and surface texture (flat, boggy, nodular). Only selected lesions were biopsied.

All therapy was performed on an outpatient basis. Initially a test area was identified. This usually measured 2–4 cm in diameter and was representative of the major portion of the PWS in color and texture. This site was chosen to allow for easy camouflage should an untoward result occur. The site was prepared with an antibacterial scrub and outlined with 2 percent tincture of brilliant green (Figure 1a and b). One percent lidocaine without epinephrine was injected for local anesthesia.

Laser vaporization of the surface was then performed using the articulated arm and handpiece of a Sharplan 733 CO_2 laser (Figure 1c). The spot size was 2 mm and power densities ranged from 498 to 796 W/cm^2; the pulse time was 0.05 sec. The pattern of vaporization was that of slightly overlapping 2-mm circles.

After the initial vaporization, the surface char was removed with a swab moistened with hydrogen peroxide. The surface was dried and then inspected with 2.5-power surgical magnifying loupes to locate any remaining vascular channels on the treated tissue bed. Such remaining vessels were selectively treated again with similar power and time factors. The procedure was discontinued when no further vessels could be identified on the surface. There was no attempt to destroy deeper vascular elements.

The bed was cleansed again and dressed with an antibiotic ointment. The patients were instructed to clean the treatment site daily and apply ointment until re-epithelialization occurred, usually at 4–6 weeks.

Patients were seen postoperatively at 4 weeks, 8 weeks, 12 weeks, and then bimonthly (Figure 1d). Test sites were evaluated for lightening and scar formation. Any patient with hypertrophic scar formation or unsatisfactory healing was eliminated from further therapy. Patients with good to excellent lightening were accepted for staged removal of the PWS (Figure 1e and f). Patients with fair to poor responses were not further treated, but were followed for possible delayed lightening of the test area.

Preliminary results

Thus far, 37 patients have been treated. All received a test procedure and follow-up as indicated. The longest follow-up is 24 months and the shortest is 8

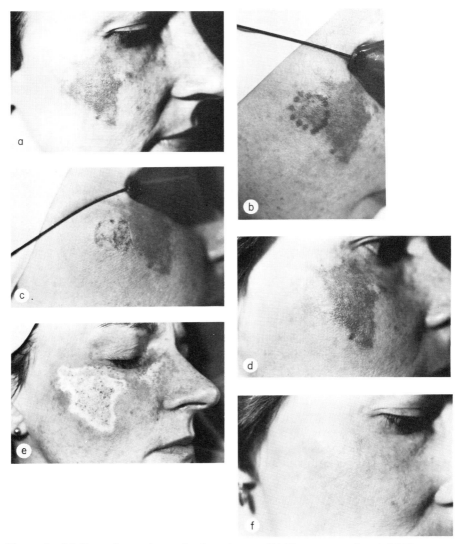

Figure 1 (*a*) Port wine stain on cheek and nose. (*b*) Test area outlined. (*c*) Test area vaporized. (*d*) Eight weeks after test. (*e*) Postoperative appearance. (*f*) Excellent result at 4 months

weeks; average follow-up time is 7 months. Three patients were lost to follow-up after the eighth week.

Twenty-one patients (57 percent) had a good to excellent response and are undergoing staged treatment (Figure 2*a–c*). Ten (27 percent) had a fair to

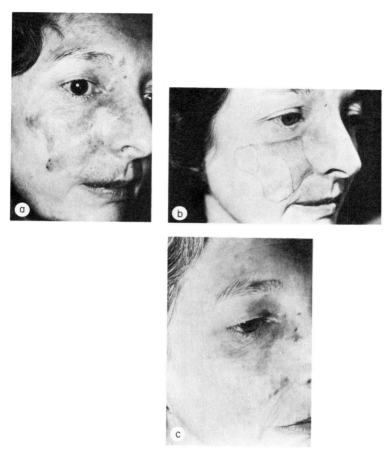

Figure 2 (*a*) Port wine stain of face. (*b*) Intermediate appearance during sequential therapy. (*c*) Good result 1 year after treatment of cheek and nose

poor response and are being followed for delayed improvement. Three of this latter group had lesions of the extremities, which are known to be more difficult to improve.

Four patients (9 percent) have developed hypertrophic scars. Three were in the test site, and of these two were on extremities (Figure 3*a–c*) and one along the mandibular angle. The fourth occurred in a patient who had had an excellent test site response but who formed excessive scar when a portion of her PWS on the midchest was treated. All these hypertrophic scars have been successfully reduced with intralesional triamcinolene acetonide injections (Figure 3*d*); all appeared by the twelfth postopertive week.

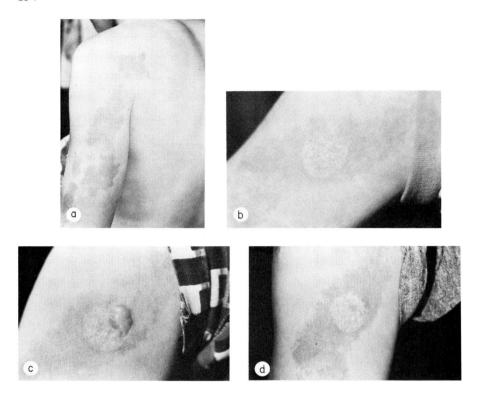

Figure 3   (*a*) Port wine stain on arm. (*b*) Test area at 4 weeks. (*c*) Hypertrophic scar at 12 weeks. (*d*) Regression of scar after intralesional steroids. Good lightening noted

Discussion

Evaluation of our early results with the CO_2 laser in comparison to results with the argon laser (our own and others' published work) has led to several preliminary conclusions. First and foremost is the fact that the CO_2 laser can be used safely and effectively in the treatment of PWS. Our data seem to corroborate the current thought that lesions of the trunk and extremities are less likely to improve than facial lesions, and that they are more likely to yield excessive unsatisfactory scarring. As with the argon laser treatment, delayed lightening of the PWS does occur in many cases and may continue for many months (up to 1 year) after therapy.

Very interestingly, a profile for predicting which PWS will improve with CO_2 laser treatment is emerging. The lesions which are light in color (pink), flat, and easily blanched on pressure seem to do best (Figure 4). This is quite fortuitous since the lesions that are most responsive to argon laser therapy are

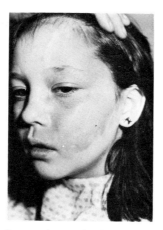

Figure 4   Type of port wine stain likely to respond to CO$_2$ laser

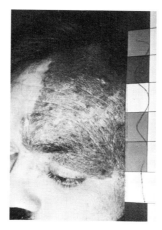

Figure 5   Type of port wine stain likely to respond to argon laser

dark (red-purple), thickened and boggy, and relatively nonblanching (Figure 5). Thus, it may be that proper preoperative selection of CO$_2$ *vs* argon laser based on the above criteria may yield uniformly better response rates.

In regard to the predictive value of biopsy specimens, we would be inclined to agree with Noe *et al.* [10] that lesions with large-caliber vessels and a high density of red blood cells are more likely to respond well to the argon laser. However, our biopsy materials have correlated so well with the above-listed clinical parameters that biopsy may prove unnecessary.

In regard to the future use of lasers to treat PWS, it may be beneficial to combine argon with CO$_2$ in a complementary sequential fashion to maximize the beneficial effect of each and minimize the negative features. Some of those studies are now in progress. Likewise, 'vessel-specific' systems may be developed to focally obliterate the ectatic lumina while sparing surrounding skin [17]. Certainly much progress has been made in the treatment of PWS and the outlook for further progress is exceedingly bright.

References

1. McBurney, E. I. Carbon dioxide laser treatment of dermatologic lesions. *South. Med. J.* 1978; **71**:795–7.
2. Kitzmiller, K. W. Laser treatment of tattoos and angiomas. *J. Med. Assoc. Ga.* 1970; **59**:385–6
3. Goldman, L., Dreffer, R. Laser treatment of extensive mixed cavernous and port-wine stains. *Arch. Dermatol.* 1977; **113**:504–5.
4. Solomon, H., Goldman, L., Henderson, B., *et al.* Histopathology of the laser treatment of port-wine lesions. *J. Invest. Dermatol.* 1968; **50**:141–6.
5. Apfelberg, D. B., Maser, M. R., Lash, H. Argon laser management of cutaneous vascular deformities. *West. J. Med.* 1976; **124**:99–101.
6. Apfelberg, D. B., Maser, M. R., Lash, H. Argon laser treatment of cutaneous vascular abnormalities: progress report. *Ann. Plast. Surg.* 1978; **1**:14–18.
7. Goldman, L. The argon laser and the port wine stain. *Plast. Reconstr. Surg.* 1980; **65**:137–9.
8. Cosman, B. Experience in the argon laser therapy of port wine stains. *Plast. Reconstr. Surg.* 1980; **65**:119–29.
9. Cosman, B. Argon laser therapy of port wine stains. *J. Med. Soc. NJ.* 1980; **77**:167–74.
10. Noe, J. M., Barsky, S. H., Geer, D. E., *et al.* Port wine stains and the response to argon laser therapy: successful treatment and the predictive role of color, age, and biopsy. *Plast. Reconstr. Surg.* 1980; **65**:130–6.
11. Apfelberg, D. B., Maser, M. R., Lash, H., *et al.* Progress report on extended clinical use of the argon laser for cutaneous lesions. *Lasers in Surgery and Medicine.* 1980; **1**:71–83.
12. Apfelberg, D. B., Greene, R. A., Maser, M. R., *et al.* Results of argon laser exposure of capillary hemangiomas of infancy—preliminary report. *Plast. Reconstr. Surg.* 1981; **67**:188–93.
13. McBurney, E. I., Leonard, G. I. Argon laser treatment of port-wine hemangiomas: clinical and histologic correlation. *South. Med. J.* 1981; **74**:925–30.
14. Apfelberg, D. B., Maser, M. R., Lash, H., *et al.* The argon laser for cutaneous lesions. *JAMA.* 1981; **245**:2073–5.
15. Ben-Bassat, M., Ben-Bassat, M., Kaplan, I. An ultrastructural study of the cut edges of skin and mucous membrane specimens excised by carbon dioxide laser. In: Kaplan, I., ed. *Laser Surgery.* Jerusalem: Academic Press, 1976:95–100.
16. Ascher, P., Ingolitsch, E., Walter, G., *et al.* Ultrastructural findings in CNS tissue with CO_2 laser. In: Kaplan, I., ed. *Laser Surgery II.* Jerusalem: Academic Press, 1976:81–5.
17. Greenwald, J., Rosen, S., Anderson, R. R., *et al.* Comparative histological studies of the tunable dye (at 577 nm) laser and argon laser: the specific vascular effects of the dye laser. *J. Invest. Dermatol.* 1981; **77**:305–10.

Cutaneous Laser Therapy: Principles and Methods
Edited by K. A. Arndt, J. M. Noe, and S. Rosen
© 1983 John Wiley & Sons Ltd

13

Modification of Lesional Skin during Argon Laser Therapy of Port Wine Stains

Barbara A. Gilchrest

The use of argon laser has revolutionized treatment of port wine stains (PWS) in the past decade. The pioneering work of Goldman and coworkers [1] was confirmed and expanded by Apfelberg and coworkers [2], who have reported (in combined series totalling 130 PWS patients) excellent results in approximately 8 percent and good results in over 50 percent. Unfortunately, in the absence of recognized risk factors for argon laser therapy, more than one in four unselected patients experienced scarring and/or poor result even at the hands of these experienced therapists. Studies by Noe and coworkers [3] provided the first data enabling the physician to advise prospective patients about the probably outcome of their therapy and to reduce the proportion of unfavorable results among selected patients. In 62 patients, favorable results correlated strongly with the interdependent variables of patient age, lesional color, fraction of dermis occupied by vessels, mean vascular area, and percent of vessels containing erythrocytes, with the latter variable providing the best single indication of response in discordant cases.

If identifiable cutaneous features indeed determine the outcome of laser therapy, in theory it would be helpful to transiently alter the lesional skin at the

137

Table 1   Possibly beneficial PWS manipulations during argon laser therapy

---

Temperature alteration
 Heating
 Chilling
Physical manipulation
 Dependency
 Tourniquet application
Pharmacologic manipulation (topical, intralesional, regional, systemic)
 Irritants
 Sympatholytics
 Anesthetics
 Prostaglandins
Reduced pigmentation
 Sunscreens
 Hydroquinone

---

time of treatment in the direction of an idealized norm. Even if causal relationships cannot be deduced from the available data, carefully evaluated, empirical modifications might still lead to improvements in laser therapy for certain patients.

Several methods by which PWS could be manipulated during argon laser therapy are shown in Table 1. Most are directed at increasing blood content of the skin, which one might predict to be helpful based on current understanding of the laser's mechanism of action (see Chapter 10). It should be noted, however, that the vessels composing a PWS may not respond to stimulae for vasoconstriction and vasodilation in the same way as vessels in the surrounding normal skin. For example, if PWS vessels respond less effectively, a vasoconstrictor may have the paradoxical effect of shunting blood into the PWS or of preventing its egress and hence of increasing hemoglobin content. Similarly, a vasodilator might result in reverse shunting or accelerated run-off of blood from the PWS and hence decreased hemoglobin content.

Attempts to evaluate the possible effect on laser therapy outcome of concurrent tourniquet application (for PWS on an extremity) or of heating lesional skin were abandoned after obtaining negative results in three patients with each modification. To date, only one modification of lesional skin has been systematically evaluated for its impact on laser therapy outcome: chilling. Because many patients volunteer that their PWS is more violaceous when they are cold, and because darker PWS are statistically associated with a better outcome [3], we undertook a study to determine whether chilling lesional skin during treatment would be beneficial [4].

Effect of chilling lesional skin

Thirty consecutive patients of the Beth Israel Hospital Laser Unit were invited

Table 2   Criteria for assessing clinical response of a PWS to argon laser therapy

		Clinical response	Color shift*	Scarring†
E	Excellent	Identical to uninvolved skin	3+	0
G	Good	Marked improvement	2+	0
			or	
			3+	1+, 2+
F	Fair	Slight improvement	1+2	0, 1+
			or	
			2+	2+
P	Poor	Undesirable result	0	0–3+
			or	
			1+	2+–3+

*Color shift in treated skin: 0, no change; 1+, slight lightening; 2+, marked lightening; 3+, identical to normal skin.

†Scarring: 0, no scar; 1+, epidermal atrophy; 2+, sclerosis, macular; 3+, hypertrophic scar.

to participate in the study, regardless of age, lesional color, site, or extent. Of 28 patients who enrolled, 23 completed the study. The average age was approximately 24 years, range 8–64 years. Fourteen were below age 21 years and only five above 36 years.

Two biopsy sites for each patient were carefully selected to be representative of the lesion overall and clinically identical to each other. One 3-mm punch biopsy was performed at room temperature (approximately 27 °C), and the other immediately after the skin surface was chilled for 2–3 minutes with an ice cube enclosed in an examining glove. Two additional representative and clinically identical 1- to 2-cm diameter sites, at least 1.0 cm distant from the biopsies, were selected as argon laser test sites. One was treated at room temperature and the other after chilling with ice exactly in the manner of the biopsy site. A Coherent Radiation Model No. 1000 argon laser with a 1.0-mm treatment aperture and 0.2-sec pulse duration was used at a setting of 1.6–1.8 W, equivalent to a power density of 200–300 W/cm^2. Each patient was treated at the same setting in both test sites. All patients were evaluated clinically by two observers after an average of 4.8 months (range 3–9 months) without reference to the treatment record or biopsy reports. Test sites were reevaluated in the same manner at each subsequent visit.

Inherent in comparisons between two treatments are objective, consistent standards for evaluation. Each test site graded excellent, good, fair, or poor according to the criteria in Table 2. Epidermal atrophy was defined as a 'cigarette paper' quality in compressed skin accompanied by increased reflectance or 'shininess' of the skin surface. In 13 of 23 patients (57 percent), the chilled site responded more favorably to laser therapy and in no instance

Table 3   Correlation between patient age, percent vascular filling in the PWS, and
outcome of argon laser therapy

Biopsy and laser therapy done at room temperature				
Clinical outcome*	E	G	F	P
Number of patients†	2	13	6	2
Patient age (years)	34.5	25.1	32.7	17.5
Percent vascular filling	13.0	26.0	24.2	7.5
Biopsy and laser therapy in chilled skin				
Clinical outcome*	E	G	F	P
Number of patients†	10	10	2	1
Patient age (years)	30.1	27.7	18	17
Percent vascular filling	36.6	30.5	0	15

*See Table 2 for definition of symbols.
†Distribution of clinical outcomes significantly better in chilled skin than in room temperature
skin ($P < 0.05$, chi sqaure analysis).

less favorably, a highly significant positive effect ($P < 0.0002$, sign test). In 11
of these 13 patients, the room temperature site manifested scarring, usually in
the form of 'epidermal atrophy', while the chilled site did not. Indeed, this
situation was observed in three additional patients whose clinical response was
nonetheless graded equal in both sites. In the remaining two cases, a more
marked color shift in the chilled skin was responsible for the better result. The
qualitative differences initially noted between the two test sites persisted in
nine of 10 patients subsequently re-evaluated after intervals of 4–18 months.

The average vascular filling in baseline lesional skin was approximately 21
percent, with chilled lesional skin approximately 6 percentage points greater
on the average. However, these relationships varied markedly among
individual patients, and values in chilled skin ranged from 51 percentage points
higher to 43 percentage points lower than in room temperture skin. Aside from
erythrocyte content of vascular lumina, there were no striking or consistent
differences in the paired biopsy specimens.

The relationship between patient age, histologic findings, and outcome of
argon laser therapy is presented in Table 3. Overall, 15 of 23 patients (65
percent) achieved a good or excellent response in the sites treated at room
temperature, and 20 of 23 (87 percent) achieved this result in the chilled
sites.

Mechanism of improvement due to chilling

It should be noted that although application of ice to the skin surface
immediately prior to use of the laser unquestionably lowers tissue temperature,
the exact degree of temperature reduction at the site of laser-beam absorption
cannot be measured and probably fluctuates during therapy. Development of a

more quantifiable and constant means of lowering skin temperture would permit more rigorous evaluation of this treatment modification and might further improve the clinical outcome of patients so treated.

The possibility of substantial irreversible damage to the epidermis and papillary dermis following argon laser therapy is apparent from histologic studies showing complete coagulative necrosis of these areas immediately after treatment [5]. Such scarring could be predicted as well from mathematical calculations utilizing a bilayer model of human skin that estimates the absorption coefficient of 488-nm–514.4-nm radiation for even a lightly melanized epidermis to be at least half that for hemoglobin [6], virtually guaranteeing tissue destruction in the area of the dermal–epidermal junction at laser doses therapeutic for dermal vascular lesions.

The original rationale for chilling the skin was the shift in PWS color from pink-red toward purple that was observed by patients when they were exposed to cold, presumably attributable to greater hemoglobin (erythrocyte) content of lesional vessels which in turn correlates with a more favorable response to the laser [3]. This hypothesis is not supported by the paired biopsy data, which show a very poor correlation between changes in percent vascular filling and clinical outcome. The data are more consistent with relative sparing of cutaneous elements such as fibroblasts and keratinocytes otherwise destroyed by heat release during laser therapy [7]. Thermodynamic models of chilled and nonchilled skin predict that reduction of heat injury during argon laser therapy should be greatest in the epidermis (D. Bourgelais, personal communication), consistent with the observed clinical findings [4]. Hence, reducing the tissue temperature may significantly widen the safety margin in laser-treated skin and so avoid scarring. Spectrophotometric readings of both PWS and normal sites suggest yet another possible mechanism, since chilling appears to affect light absorption by the skin independent of changes in hemoglobin content (S. V. Tang, B. A. Gilchrest, and D. Bourgelais, unpublished observations), perhaps through alteration of the dermal matrix.

References

1. Solomon, H., Goldman, L., Henderson, B., et al. Histopathology of the laser treatment of port wine lesions. J. Invest. Dermatol. 1968; **50**:141–6.
2. Apfelberg, D., Maser, M., Lash, H. Extended clinical use of argon laser for cutaneous lesions. Arch. Dermatol. 1979; **155**:719–21.
3. Noe, J., Barsky, S., Geer, D., et al. Port wine stain and the response to argon laser therapy: successful treatment and the predictive role of color, age, and biopsy. J. Plast. Reconstr. Surg. 1980; **65**:130–6.
4. Gilchrest, B. A., Rosen, S., Noe, J. M. Chilling port wine stains improves the response to argon laser therapy. Plast. Reconstr. Surg. 1982; **69**:278–83.
5. Apfelberg, D. B., Kosek, J., Maser, M. R., et al. Histology of port wine stains following argon laser treatment. Br. J. Plast. Surg. 1979; **32**:232–7.

6. van Gemert, M. J. C., Hulsbergen-Henning, J. P. A model approach to laser coagulation of dermal vascular lesions. *Arch. Dermatol. Res.* 1981; **270**:429–439.
7. Greenwald, J., Rosen, S., Anderson, R., *et al.* Comparative histologic studies of the tunable dye (at 577 nm) laser and argon laser: specific vascular effects of the dye laser. *J. Invest. Dermatol.* 1981; **77**:305–10.

14

Skin Healing after Argon Laser Therapy*

James L. Finley

The argon laser provides the means for delivering intense thermal energy to the abnormal vascular plexus that characterizes the port wine stain (PWS). A fraction of the incident monochromatic light is absorbed at the skin surface and is converted to thermal energy after its interaction with skin chromophores, the major one in typical Caucasian skin being hemoglobin. With the power density and pulse duration currently used, the immediate result is a diffuse superficial cautery-like necrosis histologically similar to a second-degree burn. In normal skin the depth of this process has been shown to correlate roughly with the laser power density [1]. To what degree the PWS vasculature *per se* modifies this effect is not totally understood. Histologic studies examining the acute effects of argon laser therapy on PWS [2,3] have revealed a band-like layer of necrosis involving the epidermis and superficial dermis. The necrotic zone can be demonstrated unusually well by the use of the Verhoef elastic stain (see Chapter 5). This zone of cautery (up to 0.8 mm) covers a subjacent region of heat-induced cell injury with preservation of stroma and basal lamina. The

*This work was supported by a National Center for Health Services Research grant (HS-00188), a Public Health Service Research grant (GM-00568) from the National Institutes of Health, and the American Society for Aesthetic Plastic Surgery (1980) award.

deeper portions of hair follicles, including the hair bulb and the secretory and lower exocrine portions of sweat glands, are generally too deep to be affected. The sebaceous apparatus originates in the more superficial aspects of the hair follicle and is within the field of technocausis.

Wound healing after superficial injury

Soon after injury, a minimal acute leukocytic infiltration begins peripherally. This is followed, within 24–48 hours, by epithelial regeneration from the wound margins and from adnexal structures. The exact sequence of events over the next few months regarding dermal and epidermal healing has not been examined in a systematic or quantitative manner but probably follows the patterns seen in superficial thermal or flash burns [4–6]. These studies suggest that the regenerating epithelium is laid down on top of normal-appearing dermal collagen fibers, eventually displacing the necrotic portions of epidermis and dermis. In association with the epithelial process, dermal repair proceeds through a cellular phase where polymorphonuclear leukocytes are eventually replaced by mononuclear cells. Although the neutrophil is considered important in removing bacteria and as a cell responsible for the production of degradative enzymes, it is not thought to play a direct role in fibroplasia and wound repair [7,8]. On the other hand, there is evidence that the macrophage assumes a more pivotal role in the wound healing process. *In vitro* and *in vivo* studies have shown the importance of the metabolic, growth regulatory, and secretory properties of this cell population. Activation of macrophages can occur through a variety of biologic pathways and results in a series of specialized responses including increased secretion of proteinases (collagenase, plasminogen activator, elastase, etc.), capacity to moderate cell proliferation, and the production of many biologically active molecules including interferon, endogenous pyrogens, tissue thromboplastins, prostaglandins [9], and fibronectin [10]. Activated macrophages have also experimentally shown the ability to regulate fibroblast proliferation and collagen synthesis although their precise physiologic role in this aspect of wound healing is still controversial [9].

Following and in association with the cellular phase, the first signs of fibroblast and endothelial cell proliferation occur from the viable tissue adjacent to the area of injury. Proliferative activity has also been noted in the deeper aspects of the dermis outside the area of apparent tissue injury [6]. The highly vascular and delicate granulation tissue becomes progressively organized in a process whereby the number of inflammatory cells and vessels diminishes slowly while the content of proteoglycans progressively increases. Upon this scaffold, collagen fibers are deposited and oriented. Gradually the wound changes from a cellular structure to one predominantly of collagen. Scar collagen, even 4 months after the initial injury, is metabolically more active than surrounding skin collagen and represents a dynamic equilibrium of new collagen deposition balanced against destruction and removal [11]. This process of wound healing, in the context of cutaneous laser therapy, can be influenced by a variety of factors beyond those related simply to the depth of the injury. Some of these include age, lines of skin tension, metabolic requirements, skin temperature at time of injury (see Chapter 13), medications (e.g. steroids), splinting, pressure, and the presence of old scar within the healing field.

Wound healing after argon laser therapy

In an attempt to examine the epithelial and dermal repair process after argon laser therapy, 28 patients with facial PWS were biopsied before and 4½ months after argon laser therapy [12]. In this computer-assisted study, numerous clinical and histological parameters were quantitated and compared. Pre- and post-treatment areas were assessed with a grade color chart; then scarring and color shift were combined in an overall assessment of the lesion's response to laser therapy: desirable (23 patients) or undesirable (five patients). The histologic nonvascular parameters measured (on a scale of 1 to 4+) before and after treatment included: numbers of hair follicles, sweat and sebaceous glands, epidermal thickness and degrees of parakeratosis, hyperkeratosis, melanin pigmentation, and elastosis. The characteristics of each vessel in the dermal vascular network were examined and included: number, dimensions, depth from the dermal–epidermal junction, wall thickness, and the presence or absence of luminal erythrocytes. Because of the difficulty in determining the demarcation between papillary and reticular dermis and to facilitate comparisons, the dermis was divided into 0.2-mm segments.

The post-treatment biopsies showed significant alterations in both nonvascular and vascular structures. Table 1 shows the nonvascular measurements represented as mean values before (original) and after (rebiopsy) treatment. The statistically significant changes included a slight increase in epidermal thickness and a decrease in the number of sebaceous glands without a corresponding decrease in number of hair follicles. This apparent discrepancy between sebaceous gland and hair follicle number may relate to a true decrease or it may reflect incomplete regeneration resulting in a decreased number of glands counted per section. The slight but significant increase in epidermal thickness may also relate to the stage of the regenerative process. Impressive but difficult to quantitate were the changes in dermal collagen. The rebiopsies showed considerable homogeneity, with loss of demarcation betwen papillary and reticular dermis and with fiber and bundle size being considerably reduced.

Initially, vascular measurements in the rebiopsies of the desirable and undesirable groups were compared in an attempt to determine differences in the histologic healing patterns between these subsets. No significant differ-

Table 1   Changes in nonvessel parameters after laser therapy*

	Original specimen	Rebiopsy specimen
Epidermal thickness (mm)†	0.065 ± 0.001	0.079 ± 0.003
Parakeratosis	0	0.04 ± 0.007
Hyperkeratosis	1.43 ± 0.15	1.3 ± 0.04
Elastosis	0.85 ± 0.12	1.5 ± 0.22
Melanin pigmentation	0.75 ± 0.21	1.32 ± 0.35
Hair follicles	1.79 ± 0.21	1.52 ± 0.28
Sebaceous glands†	2.89 ± 0.43	1.18 ± 0.24
Sweat glands	1.07 ± 0.18	1.48 ± 0.21

*Parakeratosis, hyperkeratosis, elastosis, melanin pigmentation graded 0 to 4+; hair follicles, sebaceous glands, and sweat glands counted; variation expressed as mean ± s.e.
†Significant at 0.01 level; Wilcoxon and *t*-tests of paired differences.
Source: Finley, J. L., Barsky, S. H., Geer, D. E., *et al.* Healing of port-wine stains after argon laser therapy. *Arch. Dermatol.* 1981; **117**:486–9. Copyright 1981, American Medical Association.

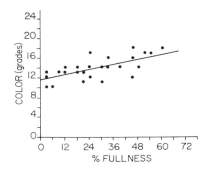

Figure 1   Relationship of color to erythrocyte-filled vessels (percent fullness). There is strong correlation between increasing color grades (pink to purple) and percent fullness (Pearson correlation coefficient = 0.69). (Reprinted with permission from *Arch. Dermatol.* 1981; **117**:486–9. Copyright 1981, American Medical Association)

ences were established and these were grouped together. The original and rebiopsy data were analyzed separately and then compared. In the original biopsies, those patients who achieved a desirable result (D) had a significantly larger vascular area, mean vessel area, and percent fullness than those with undesirable results (U). Vessel number and wall thickness were independent of therapeutic response. There was a strong correlation between percent of erythrocyte-filled vessels and color (purple lesions had many erythrocyte-filled vessels, pink lesions had few; Figure 1).

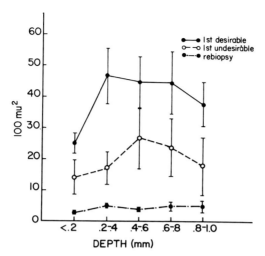

Figure 2   Mean vessel area in original biopsy specimen from those patients who achieved a desirable result after laser therapy was much greater than measurements from those who did not. Mean vessel area in repeated biopsy specimen was relatively small and showed little variation regardless of therapeutic result. Solid line indicates first desirable result; dashed line, first undesirable result; and dotted and dashed line, repeated biopsy. (Reprinted with permission from *Arch. Dermatol.* 1981; **117**:486–9. Copyright 1981, American Medical Association)

The rebiopsies showed considerable alterations in all the vessel parameters measured. The mean vessel area decreased greatly compared to the original biopsy and was significantly lower than the original (U) group (Figure 2). There was also little variability in this parameter throughout the dermis, implying a vascular network of uniform caliber and distribution. While the vascular area on rebiopsy (Figure 3) was also markedly diminished from the original (D) biopsy, it was similar to the original (U) biopsy findings and tended to decrease with increasing dermal depth. The rebiopsies contained few erythrocyte-filled vessels (Figure 4), differing markedly from original (D) biopsies and to a lesser extent from the original (U) biopsies. A similar pattern of decreasing vessel number (Figure 5) with increasing dermal depth was noted in the original and rebiopsy specimens but, paradoxically, the number of vessels at all levels trebled in the rebiopsy section. Vessel wall thickness was markedly diminished at all levels in the rebiopsies (Figuire 6).

Discussion

These data suggest that the effectiveness of argon laser therapy is based on PWS destruction and the subsequent formation of a dermis where vascular area, mean vessel area, vessel wall thickness, and the percent of erythrocyte-

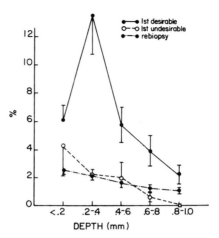

Figure 3   Vascular area (fraction of dermis occupied by vessels) in original biopsy specimen (first) from those patients who achieved a desirable result after laser therapy was high. Vascular area in repeated biopsy specimens from both therapeutic groups was considerably reduced and differed little from vascular area of patients who did not benefit from laser therapy. Solid line indicates first desirable result; dashed line, first undesirable result; and dotted and dashed line, repeated biopsy. (Reprinted with permission from *Arch. Dermatol.* 1981; **117**:486–9. Copyright 1981, American Medical Association)

filled vessels are substantially decreased even though vessel number is increased. The histologic picture is not unlike that of organized granulation tissue (Figure 7) and shows a great many similarities to the healing observed after other types of superificial thermal injuries [4,5].

The manner in which the vascular network is restored apparently alters the flow pattern and dynamics in the superficial aspects of the dermis. Numerous small, thin-walled, relatively erythrocyte-free vessels have replaced the ectatic erythrocyte-filled network. Clinically, the purple lesion of the adult becomes pink and the pink lesion of the child changes little. Why hypertrophic scarring occurs in some patients and has a predilection for certain treatment areas (perioral, angle of the jaw) is unknown.

Many patients show gradual color changes (lightening) for periods as long as 2 years after treatment. These changes in part reflect further alterations in the dermal vascular characteristics. Short-term clinical observations of treated patients suggest that the new vascular network does not undergo the progressive ectasia seen in the original lesion.

For patients who are unlikely to respond to conventional argon laser therapy, the characteristics of the incident light or the quality of absorbing chromophores might be manipulated to influence outcomes. Preliminary studies on normal skin with the tunable dye laser emitting close to one of the absorption peaks of hemoglobin have shown a selective destruction of vessels

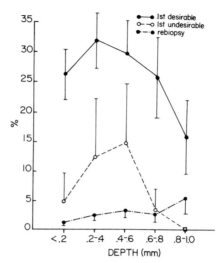

Figure 4   Percentage of erythrocyte-filled vessels was high in original biopsy specimens (first) from patients who had desirable result after laser therapy. Those who did not benefit had lower values. Overall, few erythrocyte-filled vessels were present in repeated biopsy specimens of either group. Solid line indicates first desirable result; dashed line, first undesirable result; and dotted and dashed line, repeated biopsy. (Reprinted with permission from *Arch. Dermatol.* 1981; **117**:486–9. Copyright 1981, American Medical Association)

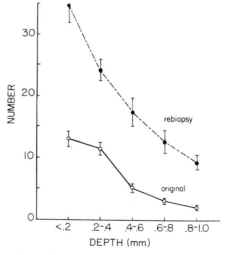

Figure 5   There were approximately three times more vessels in repeated biopsy specimens (dashed line) of both therapeutic groups than in original biopsy specimens (solid line) at all levels in dermis. (Reprinted with permission from *Arch. Dermatol.* 1981; **117**:486–9. Copyright 1981, American Medical Association)

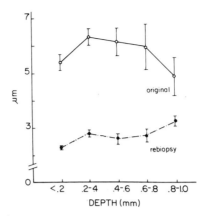

Figure 6   The vessel walls in the repeated biopsy specimens (dashed line) of both therapeutic groups were much thinner than those in original specimens (solid line) and showed much less variation. (Reprinted with permission from *Arch. Dermatol.* 1981; **117**:486–9. Copyright 1981, American Medical Association)

with preservation of adjacent dermal tissue and epidermis [1]. Attempts at altering the lesion's erythrocyte content or degree of dilatation during treatment have met with some success [13] (see Chapter 13). These methods require further scientific evaluation before their merit can be fully asessed.

Improved results might also be achieved by manipulating the healing phase after laser therapy. This has been done in an uncontrolled fashion by the use of intralesional steroids for hypertrophic scarring and by topical antibiotics, corticosteroids, and wound dressings. These and other agents that influence healing [14] may deserve closer examination, especially in the populations that respond poorly to treatment or in areas where hypertrophic scarring is a recurrent problem.

References

1. Greenwald, J., Rosen, S., Anderson, R. R., *et al.* Comparative histologic studies of the tunable dye (at 577 nm) laser and argon laser: the specific vascular effects of the dye laser. *J. Invest. Dermatol.* 1981; **77**:305–10.
2. Solomon, H., Goldman, L., Henderson, B., *et al.* Histopathology of the argon laser treatment of port-wine lesions. *J. Invest. Dermatol.*. 1968; **50**:141–6.
3. Apfelberg, D., Kosek, J., Maser, M., *et al.* Histology of portwine stains following argon laser treatment. *Br. J. Plast. Surg.* 1979; **32**:232–7.
4. Hinshaw, R., Edgar, M. Histology of healing of split thickness, full thickness autologous skin grafts and donor sites. *Arch. Surg.* 1965; **91**:658–70.
5. Hinshaw, J. R., Payne, F. W. The restoration and remodeling of the skin after a second degree burn. *Surg. Gynecol. Obstet.* 1963; **117**:732–44.

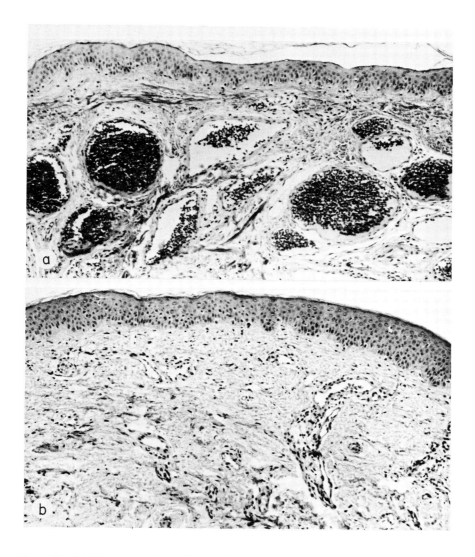

Figure 7   (a) Biopsy specimen of port wine stain taken prior to laser treatment shows typical pattern of ectatic blood-filled vessels that respond favorably to laser therapy. (b) In repeated biopsy specimen, dramatic decrease in vascular area, erythrocyte-filled vessels, and mean vessel area can be readily appreciated. Not as obvious is increased number of vessels. × 42, hematoxylin & eosin. (Reprinted with permission from *Arch. Dermatol.* 1981; **117**:486–9. Copyright 1981, American Medical Association)

6. Hinshaw, J. R., Payne, F. W. Experimental studies on the healing of radiant energy thermal burns. *Surg. Forum.* 1957; **8**:582–5.
7. Simpson, D., Ross, R. The neutrophilic leukocyte in wound repair. *J. Clin. Invest.* 1972; **51**:2009–21.
8. Diegelmann, R., Cohen, K., Kaplan, A. The role of the macrophage in wound repair: a review. *Plast. Reconstr. Surg.* 1981; **68**:107–13.
9. Leibovich, S., Ross, R. The role of the macrophage in wound repair. *Am. J. Pathol.* 1975; **78**:71–91.
10. Tsukamoto, Y., Helgel, W., Wahl, S. Macrophage production of fibronectin, a chemoattractant for fibroblasts. *J. Immunol.* 1981; **127**:673–8.
11. Madden, J. W., Peacock, E. E. Studies on the biology of collagen during wound healing. *Ann. Surg.* 1971; **174**:511–8.
12. Finleuy, J. L., BArsky, S. H., Geer, D. E., *et al.* Healing of port-wine stains after argon laser therapy. *ARch. Dermatol.* 1981; **117**:486–9.
13. Gilchrest, B. A., Rosen, S., Noe, J. M. Chilling port wine stains improves the response to argon laser therapy. *Plast. Reconstr. Surg.* 1982; **69**:278–83.
14. Madden, J. W. Wound healing: the biological basis of hand surgery. *Clin. Plast. Surg.* 1976; **3**:3–11.

Treatment of Cutaneous Lesions other than Port Wine Stains

Cutaneous Laser Therapy: Principles and Methods
Edited by K. A. Arndt, J. M. Noe, and S. Rosen
© 1983 John Wiley & Sons Ltd

15

Predicting the Utility of Argon Laser Therapy for Vascular Lesions of the Skin

Barbara A. Gilchrest and Seymour Rosen

The argon laser penetrates Caucasian human skin up to a depth of approximately 1 mm, with the usual energy levels employed during therapy [1] (see Chapter 5). Based on this knowledge of penetration depth for the laser beam, one can predict on theoretical grounds whether a given cutaneous lesion will respond favorably, if its histology is known. In many cases, these predictions have already been confirmed in clinical trials. The following sections discuss prototypic vascular lesions, other than port wine stains (PWS), and their potential responsiveness to argon laser therapy.

Strawberry hemangioma

Strawberry hemangiomas occur in 1.1–2.6 percent of infants [2,3], usually

155

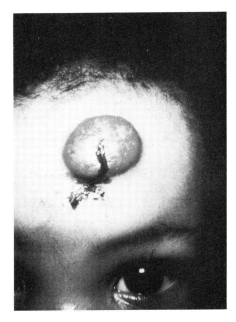

Figure 1   Strawberry hemangioma on the forehead of a 3-year-old child. Note
evidence of recent bleeding

on the face or neck. While approximately 70 percent regress spontaneously
within the first decade of life [2,3] with little or no scarring, the lesions are a
source of distress to many patients and young children (Figure 1). A few lesions
threaten vision or other critical functions.

Strawberry hemangiomas usually begin in the newborn period as pink-red
macules which rapidly evolve into red papules or plaques, and sometimes into
large masses. Lesions may be raised more than a centimeter above the
surrounding skin surface, and abnormal vessels may extend deeply into the
dermis and subcutaneous tissues in fully developed lesions [4–6].

Effectiveness of argon laser therapy has been difficult to evaluate because of
the lesion's unpredictable clinical course, but Apfelberg *et al.* have reported
improvement in three children aged 2 weeks to 13 months [7] and Dixon
has noted a beneficial response in one infant (see Chapter 17). Controlled trials
have not yet been performed.

Theoretically, the strawberry hemangiomas would be most responsive to
argon laser therapy initially, before the lesion is fully developed. Hemangiomas greater than 2 mm in depth by clinical criteria, including those that
produce the Kasabach–Merritt syndrome of platelet entrapment and subsequent bleeding diathesis [8], would not be expected to respond unless
alteration of the more superficial vessels led to involution of deeper vessels

through an indirect mechanism. All therapeutic decisions should be made with the knowledge that complete spontaneous resolution of even large lesions is common, and that current protocols for argon laser therapy are associated with a significant risk of scarring in children [9].

Cavernous hemangioma

While many authorities recognize no clear distinction between strawberry or 'capillary' hemangiomas and so-called cavernous hemangiomas, the latter term is used here to describe those lesions which typically affect the deep dermal and subcuticular vasculature, tend not to regress spontaneously, and usually present clinically as a soft, flesh-colored to purple-red nodule [10]. Larger lesions may be associated with arteriovenous fistulas, soft tissue hypertrophy and overgrowth of subjacent long bones, as in the Klippel–Trenaunay–Weber syndrome [6,11] (see Chapters 8 and 17). Cavernous hemangiomas are sometimes associated with overlying superficial vascular malformations including PWS or small papular hemangiomas.

Blue rubber bleb nevi (Figure 2) are cavernous hemangiomas affecting the skin and gastrointestinal tract. Lesions range in size up to several centimeters in diameter, may be painful, are usually multiple, and may be inherited in a dominant fashion [10,12]. We have seen such lesions with a prominent superficial component. On theoretical grounds, the deep portion of such lesions should respond very poorly to the argon laser.

Cherry hemangioma

The cherry hemangioma (De Morgan's spot) is actually an ectasia of the superficial vascular plexus (Figure 3). These bright-red dome-shaped papules are exceedingly common in middle-aged and elderly adults. Histologically, the lesion is usually confined to the upper dermis [10]. The excellent response to argon laser therapy that one would predict from this fact has been confirmed by several investigators (see Chapters 16 and 17).

Angiokeratoma

The several clinical variants of this lesion [10,13] are nearly identical histologically (Figure 4). In most instances, the vascular abnormality is confined to the papillary dermis, again predicting a favorable response to the argon laser. There are no published reports concerning laser therapy.

Pyogenic granuloma

Pyogenic granuloma is considered to be a form of benign reactive vascular

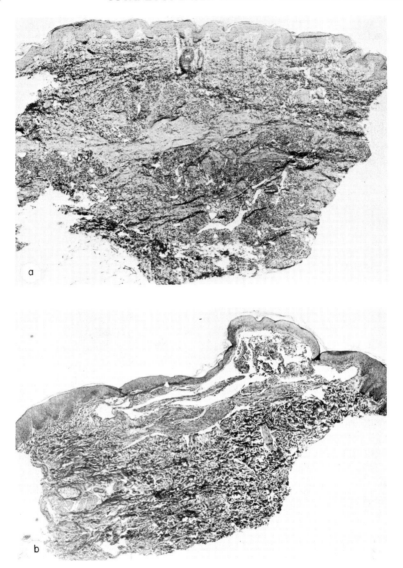

Figure 2   Blue rubber bleb nevus. These hemangiomas (a and b) may have both
           superficial and deep components. × 40, hematoxylin & eosin

hyperplasia [10]. The classic lesion arises suddenly after minor local trauma
or during pregnancy, rapidly attains its final size (usually a 10- to 100-mm^2
filiform papule), and bleeds easily (Figure 5).

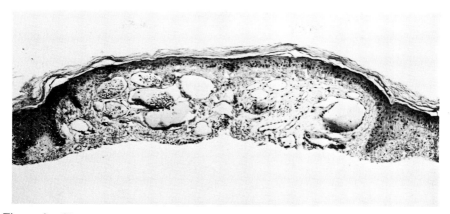

Figure 3   Cherry hemangiomas. Note the superficiality of the ectatic vessels that compose this lesion. × 90, hematoxylin & eosin

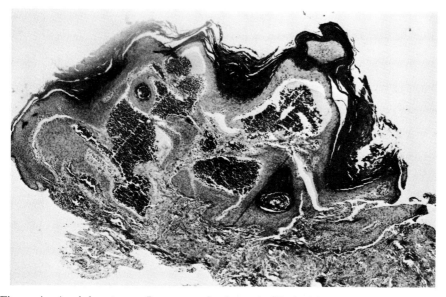

Figure 4   Angiokeratoma. Large ectatic channels filled with erythrocytes are noted closely related to hyperplastic epidermis. × 36, Masson trichrome

In theory, small pyogenic granulomas should respond well to argon laser therapy, although the attractiveness of this approach is lessened by the availability of more conventional and quite effective treatments such as electrocautery. In any case, Apfelberg and coworkers have reported excellent

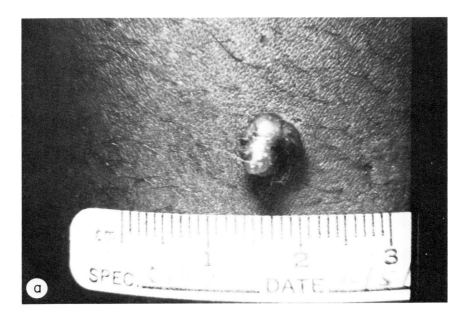

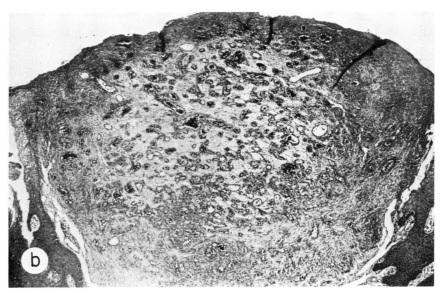

Figure 5   Pyogenic granuloma. (*a*) Typical lesion on the arm. (*b*) Histologic features include numerous small vessels associated with an edematous stroma. Note the lack of epidermis in this specimen. × 36, hematoxylin & eosin. (Clinical photograph courtesy of Sanford Goldstein, MD)

results for four pyogenic granulomas [14] and Dixon has also successfully treated such lesions (see Chapter 17). Whether the vascular papules that frequently arise in PWS after 30–50 years should be classified as pyogenic granulomas is debatable, but certainly these lesions are readily ablated with the argon laser.

Venous lakes

These asymptomatic ectasias of the superficial venular plexus are common in the elderly and classically affect the lip. On theoretical grounds, they should respond well to the argon laser, but there are no published reports.

Spider angioma

The spider angioma is an ectatic vascular lesion due to a minute, vertically disposed, arteriovenous fistula in the dermis. The central arterial punctum varies from less than 1 mm to perhaps 3 mm in diameter. Since the lesion lies predominantly in the first 1–2 mm of dermis, its good to excellent response to argon laser [15] is not surprising. Success rates are highest if the entire lesion, not just the central punctum, is treated.

Telangiectasia

Many diseases, environmental insults, and genetic factors may result in telangiectasia [10]. The involved vesels lie in the papillary and upper reticular dermis, usually within 1–2 mm of the skin surface (Figure 6). As predicted from the histologic findings, the argon laser has achieved good to excellent results with rosacea, familial hemorrhagic telangiectasia, benign nevoid telangiectasia, and radiodermatitis (see Chapters 16 and 17).

References

1. Greenwald, J., Rosen, S., Anderson, R. R., *et al*. Comparative histological studies of the tunable dye (at 577 nm) laser and argon laser: the specific vascular effects of the dye laser. *J. Invest. Dermatol.* 1981; **77**:305–10.
2. Pratt, A. G., Birthmarks in infants. *Arch. Dermatol.* 1953; **67**:302.
3. Jacobs, A. H., Walton, R. G. The incidence of birthmarks in the neonate. *Pediatrics.* 1976; **58**:218–22.
4. Bowers, R. E., Graham, E. A., Tomlinson, K. M. The natural history of the strawberry nevus. *Arch. Dermatol.* 1960; **82**:667.
5. Simpson, J. R. Natural history of cavernous haemangiomata. *Lancet.* 1959; **2**:1057–9.
6. Esterly, N. B., Solomon, L. M. Neonatal dermatology. III Pigmentary lesions and hemangiomas. *J. Pediatr.* 1972; **81**:1033–43.

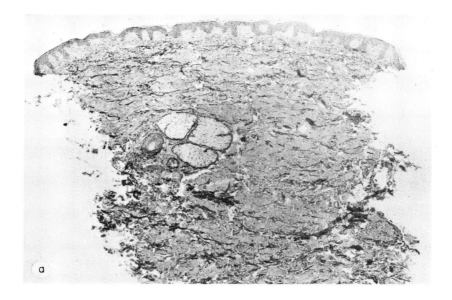

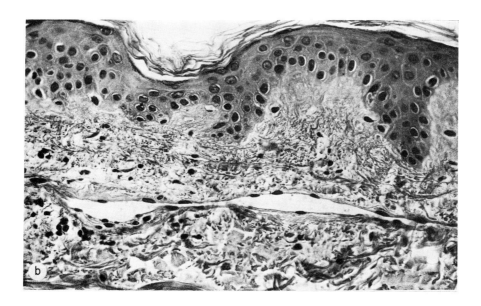

Figure 6   Essential telangiectasia. Biopsy of the skin in this condition is relatively
unremarkable. (*a*) At low power, but (*b*) at high power ectatic vessels are apparent in
the upper dermis. × 360, hematoxylin & eosin

7. Apfelberg, D. B., Greene, R. A., Maser, M. R., *et al*. Results of argon laser exposure of capillary hemangiomas of infancy—preliminary report. *Plast. Reconstr. Surg.* 1981; **67**:188–93.
8. Staub, P. W., Kessler, S., Schreiber, A., *et al*. Chronic intravascular coagulation in Kasabach–Merritt syndrome. *Arch. Intern. Med.* 1972; **129**:475–8.
9. Noe, J. M., Barsky, S. H., Geer, D. E., *et al*. Port wine stains and response to argon laser therapy: successful treatment and the predictive role of color, age, and biopsy. *Plast. Reconstr. Surg.* 1980; **65**:130–6.
10. Lever, W. F., Schaumberg-Lever, G. *Histopathology of the Skin*. Philadelphia: J. B. Lippincott, 1975.
11. Mullins, J. F., Naylor, D., Redetski, J. The Klippel–Trenaunay–Weber syndrome. *Arch. Dermatol.* 1962; **86**:202–6.
12. Fine, R. M., Derbes, V. J., Clark, W. H., Jr. Blue rubber bleb nevus. *Arch. Dermatol.* 1961; **84**:202–5.
13. Imperial, R., Helwig, E. B. Angiokeratoma. *Arch. Dermatol.* 1967; **95**:166–75.
14. Apfelberg, D. B., Maser, M. R., Lash, H., *et al*. The argon laser for cutaneous lesions. *JAMA*. 1981; **245**:2073–5.
15. Apfelberg, D. B., Maser, M. R., Lash, H. Treatment of nevi aranei by means of an argon laser. *J. Dermatol. Surg. Oncol.* 1978; **4**:172–4.

Cutaneous Laser Therapy: Principles and Methods
Edited by K. A. Arndt, J. M. Noe, and S. Rosen
© 1983 John Wiley & Sons Ltd

16

Treatment of Small Vascular and Pigmented Lesions with the Argon Laser

Kenneth A. Arndt

For more than 20 years, the argon laser has been used as a surgical tool for specific photocoagulation of a variety of cutaneous vascular and pigmented lesions [1]. The intense blue-green light of this laser (peak output at 480 nm and 514.4 nm) appears to have preferential absorption by hemoglobin (absorption peaks 420 nm, 542 nm, 577 nm) and relatively poor absorption in nonpigmented tissues. The absorbed light energy is transformed to heat, thermal damage ensues, vessels thrombose, and vascular lesions lighten or disappear.

Argon laser selectively affects red blood cell-containing vessels less than 0.5 mm in diameter that lie within the upper 1 mm of dermis, and there is relative sparing of the epidermal appendages. It is the latter characteristic that is a major distinguishing factor between simple thermal burns and laser reactions which allow healing with minimal or no scarring [2,3]. Melanocytic and other pigmented lesions also absorb laser radiation well and this characteristic too has been exploited clinically.

Laser coagulation has provided a unique tool for the treatment of port wine stains (PWS) and has become the treatment of choice for that disorder [4–7]. However, even the earliest reports on the management of cutaneous vascular lesions with the argon laser noted that numerous types of smaller vascular lesions responded well. Indeed, while treatment of PWS usually leads to a marked decrease of lesional color intensity, treatment of many smaller vascular lesions results in virtual disapperance of the vessels, often leaving no visible sequelae.

Techniques

The laser wand, which contains the terminator of the fiberoptic system transmitting light from the laser machine, is hand held at a distance of 5 cm from the skin. The pulse duration and power range I used in treating small vascular lesions was initially similar to that which had been used in previous studies of PWS therapy—irradiance 146 W/cm^2 (2.0 W, 0.2 sec, 0.1-cm spot size). This energy fluence of 29 J/cm^2 was found to be effective in eradicating lesions but appeared to be more than needed for the task. I then started using a spot size of either 0.02 cm or 0.1 cm, pulse duration kept constant at 0.2 sec and at maximal rate and power range from 0.1 W to 2.0 W (irradiance of 3.93 W/cm^2 to 7.86 W/cm^2 using the 0.02-cm spot, and 7.31 W/cm^2 to 146 W/cm^2 using the 0.1-cm spot). Varying the pulse duration and output permits administration fo the least energy necessary to ablate a lesion. The pulse duration should be the shortest available on the instrument being used (0.05 sec on the Coherent Radiation Model 1000), and the wattage setting the least which will result in visual destruction of lesions. Vessels may simply disappear leaving unaffected skin, or the overlying epidermis may become gray-white in color in response to thermal injury. The necessary power ranges from 1.0 W to 3.0 W (with a 0.05-sec pulse), and therefore allows the energy fluence to range from 3.5 J/cm^2 to 11 J/cm^2, an amount at least threefold less than previously used. Another advantage of using the shorter pulse duration is the more rapid repetition rate which allows easier tracing of small vessels. Pulses are administered in short bursts, i.e. treat for several seconds, pause for inspection of effect, then treat further as necessary for complete disappearance of lesions. It is also possible and often preferable to use a continuous beam at powers of 0.8–1.8 W (55–70 W/cm^2) for treating small lesions. The beam is carefully 'brushed' over the lesional area, taking care to steadily and continually move the beam so it does not remain focused on any one site for more than a fraction of a second. Use of the continuous beam makes it possible to blend treated areas into nontreated perilesional skin more subtly, and at this time it appears to me to be most often the method of choice.

The laser beam's diameter on the skin is another important variable. Although it might seem that smaller vessels should be treated with terminators having smaller cross-sectional openings, this is not necessarily the case (see Chapter 2). Because of the differing divergence among different terminators, the terminator with the larger aperture (0.1 cm) in the Coherent System 1000 Dermatologic Laser provides a half angle beam divergence of 0.18° while for the terminator with the smaller aperture (0.02 cm) the half angle beam divergence is 0.92° [8]. This greater divergence implies that the beam from the smaller aperture spreads much more quickly than that from the larger aperture. For distances greater than about 3.1 cm from the terminator to the skin, the laser spot size on the skin surface from the smaller aperture is actually larger than the laser spot from the larger aperture and therefore less appropriate to treat small vessels. I currently treat most patients having small vascular lesions with the 0.1-cm beam diameter, terminator-to-skin distance 3–5 cm, using continuous beam at 0.8–1.8 W, or 0.05-sec pulse duration at 1.5–3.0 W. Treatment schedules do not conform to specific diagnoses. Retreatment may take place after a 4- to 6-week interval.

Exposure of the skin to one or several pulses of laser energy produces a feeling of heat and burning but is not very painful. It is desirable to treat small lesions without anesthesia. The introduction of local anesthesia can be painful and may disrupt or temporarily obliterate the vessels to be treated. These injections not only make the lesions more difficult to visualize but may result in less intraluminal erythrocytes present to absorb the laser beam. Two percent lidocaine, a local anesthetic which causes vasodilation, is used when necessary.

Small vascular and pigmented lesions treated with the argon laser (Table 1)

The response to argon laser therapy is termed excellent if lesions completely disappear and vessels are not visible on inspection 6–12 weeks after treatment. With a good response, vessels are mostly ($\geq$ 80 percent) gone and there is marked lightening. Minimal lightening is associated with a fair response, and no change at all is considered a poor response. Adverse effects may include atrophic or hypertrophic scarring, depression of the skin surface, and hyper- or hypopigmentation. All of these improve, and some may disappear, with time (months to 1–2 years).

Rosacea, ectatic linear vessels on the nose (Figures 1 and 2)

These enlarged vessels are easily treated with the laser beam to clinical whitening, and this correlates well with continued disappearance of the vessels

Table 1   Small vascular, pigmented and hyperplastic lesions that may respond to
argon laser therapy

Vascular
  Telangiectasia
    Spider ectasia
    Actinic ectasia
    Chronic radiation dermatitis
    Associated with CRST syndrome or hereditary hemorrhagic telangiectasia
    Essential
    Nasolabial (variable response)
  Cherry angiomas
  Adenoma sebaceum
  Rosacea
    With diffuse erythema and fine ectasia
    With linear ectatic vessels on nose
  Pyogenic granuloma
  Capillary hemangiomas (strawberry hemangiomas) of infancy*
Pigmented
  Tattoos
    Decorative
    Traumatic
  Melanocytic
    Café-au-lait
    Lentigines
    Nevi
    Giant hairy nevus†
    Lentigo maligna
    Dermal melanocytosis (nevus of Ota)
Hyperplastic†
  Fibrous papule
  Rhinophyma
  Seborrheic keratosis

*See Chapter 17.
†See [7].

after healing. In some patients a slight depression in the skin's surface can be
seen on examination with oblique lighting 1–3 months later. This appears to
represent the space previously occupied by the now-destroyed vascular area,
but may also reflect some epidermal and upper dermal atrophy. Of the first
eight patients I have treated, four showed excellent results, three good and one
fair results [9].

Diffuse erythema and ectasia of the nose (Figure 3)

Diffuse redness of the nose with multiple minute ectatic vessels is seen in
patients with rosacea or in a small number of individuals who are post-rhinoplasty or other operative or nonoperative trauma to the nose. It is possible to

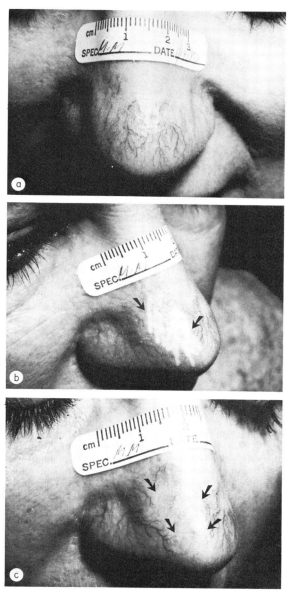

Figure 1 Rosacea ectatic vessels. (*a*) Before treatment. (*b*) Immediately after treatment. (*c*) Twelve
weeks later. Vessels are almost completely absent in
treated area (between arrows). (From *Arch. Dermatol.* 1982; **118**:220–4. Copyright 1982, American
Medical Association)

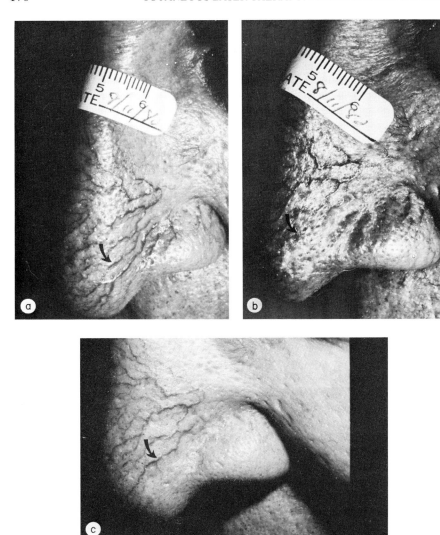

Figure 2   Rosacea, ectatic vessels. (*a*) Before treatment. All vessels below that noted by *arrow* were treated. (*b*) Immediately after treatment. (*c*) Eight weeks later. All vessels below that noted by *arrow* were treated. (From *Arch. Dermatol.* 1982; **118**:220–4. Copyright 1982, American Medical Association

totally eliminate all these superficial vessels with argon laser therapy. The vessels are so small that it is impossible to eliminate them individually and the entire area must be treated. This was clearly evident in a test spot on one

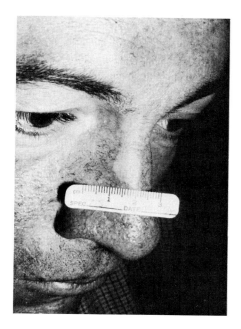

Figure 3   Rosacea, diffuse ectasia. Test site 8 weeks after treatment. All vessels are absent in test site. (From *Arch. Dermatol.* 1982; **118**:220–4. Copyright 1982, American Medical Association)

treated patient when viewed 5 months after therapy [9]. Apfelberg *et al.*[7] reported good results in 3/3 patients with acne rosacea, and Noe *et al.* have defined the post-rhinoplasty 'red nose' syndrome (Figure 4) and described its successful treatment in one patient [10].

Spider ectasia

The response of spider ectatic lesions (nevi aranei) to the argon laser is nearly always excellent (Figure 5). Few pulses (usually 10–60) are needed to induce whitening or disappearance of lesions, and this clinical change is always followed by continued absence of lesions after healing. 'Brushing' the entire area with the continuous laser beam is at times more effective than trying to trace each individual vessel. Slight hypopigmentation and atrophy are occasionally sequelae. Of seven patients treated, five showed excellent results and two good results. Three of these seven patients had previously noted recurrence after two to seven electrosurgical treatments and none has recurred after laser treatment [9].

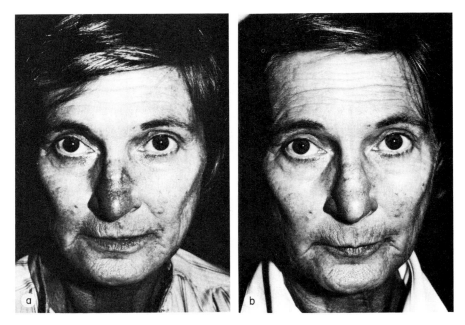

Figure 4 Postrhinoplasty 'red nose'. (*a*) Before treatment, 27 weeks after rhinoplasty. (*b*) Four weeks later. (From Noe, J. M., Finley, J., Rosen, S., *et al*. Postrhinoplasty 'red nose': differential diagnosis and treatment by laser. *Plast. Reconstr. Surg.* 1981; **67**:661–4)

Telangiectasia of various causes

Ectatic vessels of various etiologies generally respond well to the argon laser. These include lesions induced by actinic damage, chronic radiation dermatitis associated with the CRST syndrome (systemic sclerosis) or hereditary hemorrhagic telangiectasia, essential telangiectasia consisting of mats of isolated small vessels (Figures 6 and 7), and nasolabial telangiectasia. The latter site should be treated with special care as it is more at risk for atrophy. Lesions on the face and neck respond best, and those on the lower extremities do least well, as described below. Apfelberg *et al.*[6] have treated 53 patients with telangiectasia with 47 excellent results, four good and two poor.

Adenoma sebaceum of tuberous sclerosis (Figure 8)

One 13-year-old boy with hundreds of bright-red elevated lesions of adenoma sebaceum (angiofibromas) on the face and nose has been treated with strikingly positive results [11]. Lesions disappeared entirely and no atrophy

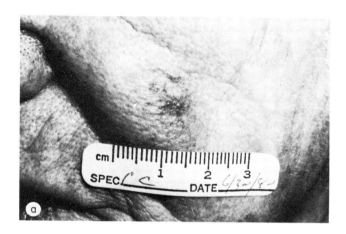

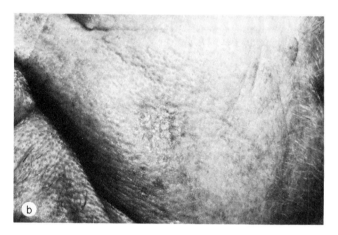

Figure 5 Spider ectasia recurrent after six electrosurgical treatments. (*a*) Before treatment. (*b*) Six weeks later. (From *Arch. Dermatol.* 1982; **118**:220–4. Copyright 1982, American Medical Association)

ensued. Some new flesh-colored and pink papules have appeared over the subsequent 2 years.

Cherry hemangiomas (Figure 9)

These common lesions, also referred to as senile angiomas or De Morgan's spots, respond in uniformly excellent fashion. This was seen in 2/2 of my patients [9] and 5/5 reported by Apfelberg *et al.*[7].

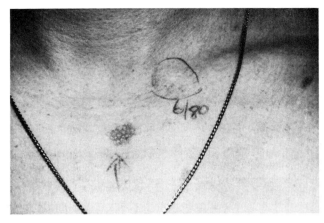

Figure 6   Essential telangiectasia. *Arrow*: untreated lesion. *Circle*: lesion treated 9 months before

Superficial leg vessels

Ectatic vessels on the lower leg do *not* respond well to laser radiation. These lesions consist of very fine networks of small superficial purple vessels, or others which are larger, deeper, more linear, and blue in color. These poor results have been noted by Goldman (see Chapter 21), Apfelberg *et al.*[7], and Dixon (see Chapter 17) as well. Of eight patients I have treated, two had excellent results, one good, two poor, and three adverse (some vessels more prominent, intermittent vessel loss (staccato type), hyperpigmentation and atrophy) [9]. The lack of desirable results may be related to the small vessel diameter or deeper location in the skin, less adequate healing on the lower extremities, or the use of nonoptimal laser power densities or techniques.

Pigmented lesions

Melanin is the major absorber of light in the epidermis from the UVB spectrum through the visible to the near-infrared (320–1000 nm). Longer wavelengths are absorbed less well and penetrate more easily through the epidermis. Deeply pigmented persons are therefore not good candidates for argon laser therapy because of possible pigment cell destruction and subsequent hypopigmentation. However, epidermal and dermal melanocytic and other pigmented lesions do absorb laser radiation well and this characteristic can be used to advantage. Apfelberg *et al.*[7] describe successful treatment of five patients with melanocytic nevi, one with a café-au-lait spot, one with actinic lentigines ('liver spots'), one test area within a giant hairy nevus, and three patients with

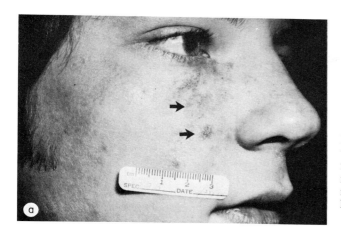

Figure 7 Essential telangiectasia. (*a*) Before treatment. (*b*) Immediately after treatment. (*c*) Ten months later. Area treated is noted by *arrows*

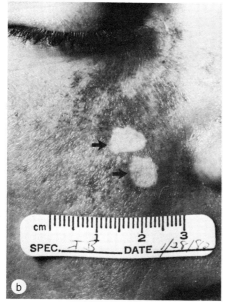

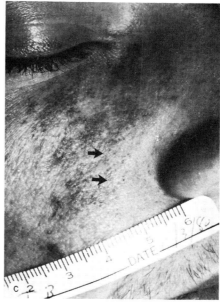

seborrheic keratoses. They noted good results in two patients with nevus of Ota and poor results in one. Good results have been attained in our laboratory after treatment of multiple nevi on one patient, complete depigmentation but with some atrophy on another patient with a large lower-extremity café-au-lait spot, good results in several patients with forearm and dorsal hand lentigines, and complete disapperance of a large lentigo maligna on the bridge of the nose of a 45-year-old man, leaving only minimal epidermal atrophy. It is mandatory

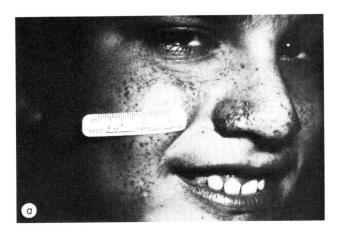

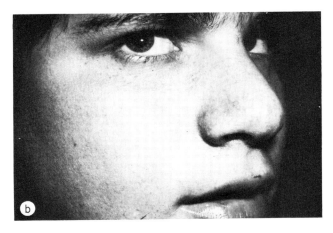

Figure 8   Adenoma sebaceum. (*a*) Before treatment. (*b*) One year after treatment to entire face. Some small untreated skin-colored lesions remain. (From Arndt, K. A. Adenoma sebaceum. Successful response to argon laser. *Plast. Reconstr. Surg.* 1982;) **70**:91–93

to have good clinical, and if necessary histologic, evidence concerning the nature of pigmented melanocytic lesions prior to treatment. The effect of argon laser extends only 0.5–1.0 mm into the skin. Although this may be adequate for benign lesions and may be sometimes the treatment of choice for superficial atypical lesions such as lentigo maligna, it is inappropriate for truly malignant lesions. Cells deeper than 1 mm or those extending down follicular structures will not be destroyed. Careful follow-up of patients with laser-treated melanocytic lesions is important.

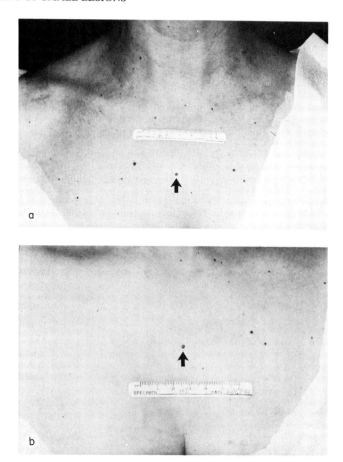

Figure 9   Cherry hemangioma. (*a*) Before treatment. All lesions to the patient's right (reader's left) of midsternal hemangioma shown by *arrow* were treated. (*b*) Six weeks later. (From *Arch. Dermatol.* 1982; **118**:220–4. Copyright 1982, American Medical Association)

Comment

The argon laser is capable of destroying enlarged or ectatic superficial vessels present in many types of lesions. Those abnormalities that respond most easily and show a good cosmetic result consist of larger vessels or confluent mats and have an intense and deep red-blue color (spider ectasia, rosacea with ectatic long vessels, cherry angiomas, post-rhinoplasty 'red nose', adenoma sebaceum). Vascular lesions that tend to do less well contain very fine vessels or are located on the lower extremities. When vessel size is minute so that little intraluminal hemoglobin is present to absorb the laser radiation, the surrounding skin is often more severely damaged and this may lead to atrophy. Using the minimum pulse duration and energy necessary to destroy vessels should help lower the incidence of adverse effects.

Alternative methods exist for treating many of these lesions. Cryosurgery with liquid nitrogen can effect useful changes in some angiomas but this treatment method is not useful for smaller vascular lesions. Injection with sclerosing agents may occasionally be beneficial in ectatic leg vessels, but the small size of most vessels makes this technique difficult, and there is no ideal sclerosing solution available. Delivery of thermal energy by electrolysis, electrosurgery with an epilating needle, or cautery, if carefully performed, should result in equally good results with many lesions of the type discussed in this chapter.

Thus far the reports of usefulness of argon lasers for pigmented lesions are only anecdotal. The appropriate use of various types of laser radiation for benign and malignant melanocytic lesions needs comprehensive and detailed study. The optimal techniques of argon laser use for all lesions with regard to spot size of laser light, power density, pulse duration, and distance of fiberoptic terminator from skin must still be defined.

References

1. Arndt, K. A., Noe, J. M. Lasers in dermatology. *Arch. Dermatol.* 1982; **118**:293–5.
2. Apfelberg, D., Kosek, J., Maser, M. R., *et al.* Histopathology of port wine stains following argon laser treatment. *Br. J. Plast. Surg.* 1979; **32**:232–7.
3. Finley, J. L., Barsky, S., Geer, D., *et al.* Healing of port wine stains after argon laser therapy. *Arch. Dermatol.* 1981; **117**:486–9.
4. Cosman, B., Experience in the argon laser therapy of port wine stains. *Plast. Reconstr. Surg.* 1980; **65**:119–29.
5. Noe, J. M., Barsky, S. H., Geer, D. H., *et al.* Port wine stains and the response to argon laser therapy: successful treatment and the predictive role of color, age, and biopsy. *Plast. Reconstr. Surg.* 1980; **65**:130–6.
6. Apfelberg, D. B., Maser, M. R., Lash, H., *et al.* Progress report on extended clinical use of the argon laser for cutaneous lesions. *Lasers in Surgery and Medicine.* 1980; **1**:71–83.
7. Apfelberg, D. B., Maser, M. R., Lash, H., *et al.* The argon laser for cutaneous lesions. *JAMA.* 1981; **245**:2073–5.
8. Arndt, K. A., Noe, J. M., Northam, D. B. C., *et al.* Laser therapy. Basic concepts and nomenclature. *J. Am. Acad. Dermatol.* 1981; **5**:649–54.
9. Arndt, K. A. Argon laser therapy of small cutaneous vascular lesions. *Arch Dermatol.* 1982; **118**:220–4.
10. Noe, J. M., Finley, J., Rosen, S., *et al.* Postrhinoplasy 'red nose': differential diagnosis and treatment by laser. *Plast. Reconstr. Surg.* 1981; **67**:661–4.
11. Arndt, K. A. Adenoma sebaceum. Successful response to argon laser. *Plast. Reconstr. Surg.* 1982; **70**:91–93.

Cutaneous Laser Therapy: Principles and Methods
Edited by K. A. Arndt, J. M. Noe, and S. Rosen
© 1983 John Wiley & Sons Ltd

17

Treatment of Other Selected Vascular Cutaneous Lesions with the Argon Laser

John A. Dixon

The successful use of the argon laser in the treatment of port wine stains (PWS) has aroused interest in the use of this treatment modality in patients with a broad spectrum of cutaneous vascular problems [1–4]. Because of the complex nature of the blood supply of the skin, these lesions represent a broad range of venous, arterial, mixed arteriovenous, superficial, and deep processes. Consistent with this range of presentation, the impact of the lesions upon the patient ranges from almost frivolous and cosmetic to disabling and life-threatening.

Because of the variety of lesions, selection criteria are almost nonexistent. As with PWS, however, superficial lesions respond better than deep lesions. Lesions of the deep red/blue/purple hues generally respond better than do those of light pink to pale red hues.

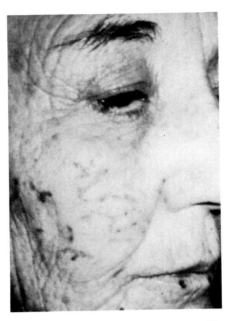

Figure 1   Osler–Weber–Rendu disease. Extensive lesions of branching configuration
on skin, tongue, nasal and gastric mucosa

These lesions vary from about capillary size to 1- to 2-mm vessels, and
therefore the irradiance (power density) required for photocoagulation may
range from 20 to 140 W/cm^2. As with PWS, the operator should start with a
low power setting (0.8 W) and a short application time (0.2 sec), test a spot,
then gradually increase watts or time of application until the desired
coagulation of the vessel is obtained with minimal superficial cutaneous injury.
The continuous technique is usually preferable with these discrete, linear,
punctate, or channeled lesions.

Osler–Weber–Rendu disease (hereditary hemorrhagic telangiectasia)

This hereditary disorder may present with lesions of the tongue, lips, skin,
nasal or gastrointestinal mucosa. The cutaneous vascular lesions present in
three general fashions. Punctae are the most common and occur in the skin and
mucous membranes. They may be slightly raised and are seen on the fingers,
face, lips, or nasal mucous membranes. The other two varieties have either a
spider or branched configuration. A typical example of patient with
Osler–Weber–Rendu disease of the branchial configuration is seen in Figure 1.
Diagnosis is dependent upon the identification of the characteristic lesion in
addition to a familial tendency in which the disease is inherited as a simple

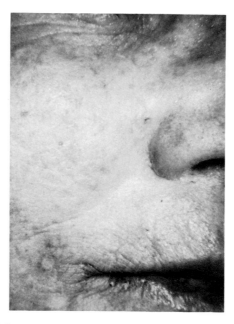

Figure 2   Osler–Weber–Rendu disease 6 months following argon laser treatment. Good vessel obliteration. No scarring. Minimal hypopigmentation

Mendelian autosomal dominant trait. In addition to their skin lesions, bleeding from the nasal mucosa as well as lesions in the gastrointestinal tract have attracted a number of these patients to the argon laser hemostasis program.

Treatment has been carried out with 1.5–2.0 W continuous application of argon laser radiation and 2-mm spot size. Similar results may be obtained with 1.0–1.5 W intermittent application of 0.2-sec duration. The continuous application seems easier due to the ability to follow the linear branched telangiectases. Treatment is carried to a blanching of the vessel with no more than whitening of the overlying skin. The result of such a treatment is seen in Figure 2.

The patients with these lesions of the skin have been treated with excellent results. No scarring has been noted. In the lesions of the mucosa of the nose and gastrointestinal tract, an inexorable progression of these lesions has occurred, necessitating 'harvesting' the vascular abnormalities when they become large, bleeding, or ulcerative. In these areas, multiple lesions have been coagulated, bleeding controlled, and sites of treatment mapped. When bleeding recurs months later, it is possible to identify the scarred blanched areas of previous treatment. New vascular bleeding lesions are now evident [5]. The longest observation of any of these patients is now only 3 years, yet no recurrence or

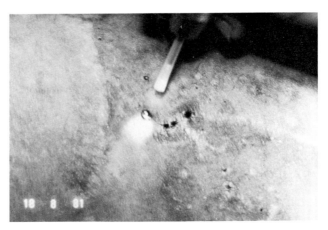

Figure 3   Klippel–Trenaunay–Weber syndrome of the leg. Scars from previous surgical excision. Laser coagulation of superficial bleeding venous lakes

progression of skin lesions has been noted similar to that present in nasal or gastric mucosa.

Klippel–Trenaunay–Weber syndrome (osteohypertrophic angioectasia)

Patients with this syndrome present gross hypertrophy of the extremities or digits with large dilated subcutaneous veins and purplish cutaneous lesions with small punctate dark angiomatous nodules that are subject to trauma and bleeding [6]. Obviously, it is impossible to treat deep vascular lesions with the argon laser because of depth of penetration and size of vessels involved. The small punctate bleeding nodules, however, have been very successfully managed using argon laser photocoagulation such as seen in Figure 3. Treatment is usually carried out without local anesthesia as this tends to distort the punctuate lesions and reduce the efficacy of coagulation. Using power settings of 1.5–2.0 W, a spot application of 0.2–0.4 sec is usually well tolerated by these patients. In larger vessels, more power may be required. If the laser fiber is placed too close to the lesion (smaller spot size, high laser irradiance), vaporization of the vessel walls and bleeding will occur. It is best to start holding the laser stylus 3–4 cm away from the skin, test a representative spot, then gradually move in closer so that the vesels may be treated, go into spasm, and be coagulated prior to receiving sudden high irradiance with possible ensuing rupture.

Pyogenic granuloma

Pyogenic granuloma is a local, superficial, and often ulcerated polypoid lesion composed of newly formed capillaries in an edematous matrix. These may occur at any age and in either sex, on the palm of the hands, fingers, scalp, or lips. Histologic section reveals a nodular collection of lymphocytes associated with hyperplasia of blood vessels. Numerous red blood cells are usually present, with occasional dense nodules of lymphocytes surrounding blood vessels. Despite the implication of infectious cause implied by its name, proof of this etiology is lacking. Apfelberg *et al.* have treated four of these lesions with excellent results [3]. Successful treatment has been carried out on such lesions arising in PWS in the scalp, hand, the margin of an eyelid, and angle of the mouth. Inability to treat between the teeth resulted in failure of therapy to a gingival pyogenic granuloma between the central and lateral incisor teeth. This lesion eventually required surgical excision.

It is interesting that some of these lesions, especially those occuring in PWS following laser therapy, may have varying amounts of vascular and fibrous tissue. The vascular lesions may be easily coagulated. It may be difficult to entirely coagulate the larger ones with a greater fibrous component. In these lesions, it is useful to coagulate the lesions in a circumferential fashion with the laser, excise the nodule flush with the skin with a scalpel, then coagulate the base with the laser.

Essential telangiectasia (spider veins, intracutaneous varices, sunburst veins, small varicose veins of the legs)

These superficial dilated veins begin to appear in women in their early twenties and progress through the late forties and fifties. Although referred to as 'varicose veins', they probably have no relationship to true varicosities. Although occasionally a 'burst' will appear around a central vein, frequently the branching veins appear to be discontinuous without central collecting systems. Many women regard them as unsightly, preventing them from wearing tennis shorts, bathing suits, etc., and have a really desperate desire for removal of these lesions.

Treatment with the argon laser has consisted of continuous application of 1.5–2.0 W argon laser, 2-mm spot size, tracing out each individual vein until it blanches. The skin color over the treated veins should be white, not gray or black, following treatment. Minimal postoperative pain with only occasional itching is noted. Because of re-epithelialization with resultant healing at the sites of coagulation, it is necessary to wait 3–6 months to determine results following treatment.

For small areas of involvement, intradermal field block with 4 percent prilocaine provides adequate anesthesia. Infiltration into the telangiectatic area discolors and obliterates the veins, making coagulation difficult. Many patients will tolerate brief periods of coagulation of these vessels without anesthesia. This has to be evaluated very carefully on an individual basis, however. If, after 3 months, an initial 1–1.5 square inch test area looks promising, treatment of larger areas may be carried out under local anesthesia, or general anesthesia in patients with extensive involvement.

The evaluation and treatment of these patients is among the most vexing in our laser treatment experience. These patients are usually extremely conscious of their apperance; hence, their expectations are high and tolerance for postlaser pigmentation, depigmentation, or scarring is low.

Apfelberg *et al.* have reported poor results in a series of 13 such patients [1]. Our results are as follows:

Essential telangiectasia	
No. of patients	25
Excellent result	0
Good result	53%
Fair result	0
Poor result	48%
Scarring	4%

Although the original group of patients is still being observed and occasional patches or touch-up areas treated, we are very ambivalent about this application of the laser. Some improvement does seem to occur. Some treated veins will appear 'beaded' with areas of obliteration and depression interspersed with areas of obviously patent veins. Scarring occurred in one patient in the area behind and below the knee. While this appears to be an area particularly exposed to irritation and trauma, the patient also had a history of keloid formation that was not adequately identified prior to treatment.

It is our feeling that a wavelength that would provide greater absorption of hemoglobin by the laser with less epidermal and dermal injury might make this an effective form of treatment. Results at this time could only be described as equivocal at best. No new patients are being added to the study group for the present. Rotering's study indicated that 58 percent of our patients did not feel the results justified the expense, effort, and hazard of therapy (R. H. Rotering, personal communication).

Lymphangioendothelioma

Five lesions have been encountered that appear to be predominantly lymphangiomatous albeit with some hemangiomatous component. The argon laser has not proved useful in the treatment of clear, watery vesicles of the lymphangioma. Where bluish-red blebs are present in association with the lymphangioma, superficial argon laser therapy may be helpful. In some such cases, electrodesiccation of the clear blebs has given some superficial improvement in the appearance of the lesions. The CO_2 laser has been used successfully in some of these tumors.

Capillary hemangiomas of infancy

Frequent calls are received (almost from the delivery room) from the distressed parents of infants with strawberry hemangiomas or capillary hemangiomas of infancy. As described by Bowers *et al.* [7] and others, 50 percent of these will resolve by age 5 and 70 percent by age 7 years. Management has generally revolved around the expectation of involution and avoidance of trauma or scarring due to unwise intervention. The families of patients with this problem are reassured and urged to adopt a policy of observation. In unusual cases, however, lesions may bleed, be in an area subjected to trauma and ulceration, or the lesion may be on the eyelid or nose where cartilage may be deformed. Hemangiomas of the mouth or oral cavity might interfere with feeding, or those of the genital area block bladder or bowel function. Apfelberg *et al.* have recently reported successful treatment of infants with bleeding hemangiomas of the cheek, medial calf, and nasal alar regions with the argon laser [3]. We have successfully treated one infant with a capillary hemangioma of the gluteal fold that had become ulcerated, infected, and bled. It should be emphasized that argon laser treatment of these lesions should be undertaken only for very specific indications, not generally applied to what is usually a self-limited process.

Malignant hemangioendothelioma

One patient with multiple ulcerated cutaneous metastases from a malignant hemangioendothelioma has been treated symptomatically at the request of the oncologists. These lesions are purplish-red, highly vascular, both intracutaneous and subcutaneous, and associated with ulceration and bleeding. Using 2.0 W argon laser continuous to a point of vascular blanching, it was possible to reduce the size and control the bleeding and ulceration from these lesions for a period of 4 months prior to the patient's death.

References

1. Apfelberg, D. B., Maser, M. R., Lash, H. Argon laser treatment of cutaneous vascular abnormalities. *Ann. Plast. Surg.* 1978; **1**:14–18.
2. Apfelberg, D. B., Greene, R. A., Maser, M. R., *et al.* Results of argon laser exposure of capillary hemangiomas of infancy—preliminary reports. *Plast. Reconstr. Surg.* 1981; **67**:188–93.
3. Apfelberg, D. B., Maser, M. R., Lash, H., *et al.* The argon laser for cutaneous lesions. *JAMA.* 1981; **245**:2073–5.

4. Arndt, K. A. Argon laser therapy of small cutaneous vascular lesions. *Arch. Dermatol.* 1982; **118**:220–4.
5. Parkin, J. L., Dixon, J. A. Laser photocoagulation in hereditary hemorrhagic telangiectasia. *Otolaryngol. Head Neck Surg.* 1981; **98**:204–8.
6. Gaidawich, I. F., Campanacci, M. Vascular haematomata and infantile angioectatic osteohyperplasia of the extremities. *J. Bone Joint Surg. [Am]*. 1962; **44**:815–42.
7. Bowers, R. E., Graham, E. A., Tomlinsen, J. M. The natural history of the strawberry nevus. *Arch. Dermatol.* 1960; **82**:59–72.

Cutaneous Laser Therapy: Principles and Methods
Edited by K. A. Arndt, J. M. Noe, and S. Rosen
© 1983 John Wiley & Sons Ltd

18

Use of the CO_2 Laser for Non-PWS Cutaneous Lesions

Philip L. Bailin

The carbon dioxide (CO_2) laser has been utilized in surgery for several years. Many disciplines have found it advantageous; these include otolaryngology, plastic surgery, gynecology, general surgery, and neurosurgery. Each of these has developed relative indications for use of the laser, and even some absolute indications have been identified (e.g. surgery on the hemophiliac patient).

The application of the CO_2 laser to dermatologic surgery has been reported by several authors (1–12), most frequently in treatment of tattoos and port wine stains (PWS). Since dermatology is primarily an outpatient office-based specialty, few dermatologists have had access to these lasers which are of relatively high cost and, for the most part, located in hospital operative facilities.

The purpose of this chapter is to briefly describe and comment on our experience with the CO_2 laser in general dermatologic surgery. Since January 1980, we have performed 211 CO_2 laser surgical procedures in our laser unit.

This unit is located in the outpatient clinic of the Dermatology Department, Cleveland Clinic Foundation. Thus, all procedures were performed on ambulatory patients under local anesthesia—conditions comparable to an office environment.

The instrument utilized was the Sharplan 733 CO_2 laser manufactured in Israel. This laser is equipped with an articulated arm system through which the laser radiation is channeled to a surgical handpiece. The invisible beam is aimed precisely by means of coaxial, highly visible, red helium–neon low-energy laser aiming beam. No integrated operating microscope was present on this unit, and it is felt that the microscope is nonessential for dermatologic surgery. The articulated arm–handpiece configuration is far more flexible and practical for such applications.

Aspects of CO_2 physics and optical properties are discussed in Chapters 2 and 12. Certain features of this laser make it highly and uniquely desirable for skin surgery. These features should be reviewed.

The CO_2 laser emits invisible far-infrared radiation of 10,600-nm wavelength. This radiation is totally absorbed in a depth of only 0.1–0.2 nm of water. Cutaneous tissue has a similar coefficient of absorption since it is 85–90 percent water. The internal scatter of the laser beam in water (tissue) is minimal (< 3 percent). These two factors, low penetration and minimal scatter, make the CO_2 laser a highly *localized* tissue-destructive modality.

The CO_2 laser is a continuous wave rather than pusle wave type of laser. This means that radiation energy is continuously produced by the laser tube as long as electrical pumping energy is supplied. Therefore, a continuous radiation beam of uniform energy (without pulse peaks and valleys) is available for tissue application. This means that effects on tissue are regular and nonvarying. Pulse wave types of lasers, on the contrary, build energy within the lasing medium, discharge laser radiation at a peak, then require a brief resting period while energy builds again. This results in a varying intensity of radiation periodically reaching the target tissue. Such pulsed irradiation may cause uneven tissue damage and there is a theoretical potential for malignant cell survival and dislodgement from the target site.

It must not be surmised from the preceding that the radiation beam of the CO_2 laser cannot be applied to tissue in a pulsed or intermittent fashion. This can very readily be accomplished by interposing a shutter system, either mechanical or electro-optical, in the path of the beam, much like in a camera. However, this shutter merely opens or closes an exit port but does nothing to the character of the beam. It is still a continuous wave of steady uniform output as described above.

The CO_2 laser radiation is of such a wavelength (far-infrared) that it cannot presently be transmitted through an optical fiber system. Therefore, transmission is through articulated sealed tubes via angled mirror joints. The radiation finally reaches a lightweight, freely movable surgical handpiece containing a focusing lens. The instrument may be fitted with handpieces of various focal lengths. Those currently available are in the range of 50–125 m focal length. This yields a *focused* treatment spot size on the target tissue of 0.1–0.2 mm diameter. If the power output is in the range of 15–25 W, the power density (power/area) would be in the range of 50,000–80,000 W/cm². If the beam is *defocused* by moving the handpiece away from the tissue, the spot size enlarges to a diameter of approximately 2.0 mm. At the same power output of 15–25 W, the power density would be in the range of 500–1000 W/cm². The significance of this will be explained shortly.

When the laser radiation impacts on skin tissue, the result is the instantaneous conversion of intracellular and extracellular water to tissue steam at a temperature of 100 °C. This instantaneous reaction is called vaporization. It results in instantaneous cellular destruction. Because this phenomenon occurs so very rapidly, there is minimal thermal energy transmission to adjacent cells [13]. This yields an extremely localized area of tissue destruction in which the immediately adjacent tissue is virtually unaffected. This differs greatly from other forms of thermal destruction (cautery, high-frequency current, cryosurgery) in which destruction shows a central maximum zone and a gradually decreasing peripheral gradient.

Such focal destructive capability, when utilized in a focused mode (impact spot of only 0.1–0.2 mm), can be equivalent to an incisional scalpel cut. Conversely, if the beam is defocused to an impact spot of 2.0 mm with resultant lower-power density, a surface may be rapidly vaporized away in an 'airbrush' fashion. Both occur without damage to adjacent or underlying tissue. This amazing versatility makes the CO₂ laser uniquely valuable for dermatologic surgical application.

Furthermore, the CO₂ laser possesses other features of great value in cutaneous surgery. In the focused incisional mode (high-power density; small spot size) blood vessels up to 0.5 mm in caliber are instantly sealed as they are cut, leading to virtually bloodless surgery. If larger vessels are severed (up to 1.5 mm caliber), they may be sealed by grasping the end with a forceps and lasing the severed end with the defocused beam (low-power density; larger spot size). Additionally, lymphatics are sealed as the laser cuts through or vaporizes tissue, leading theoretically to a diminished risk of metastasis in malignant lesions. The CO₂ beam also sterilizes as it cuts, minimizing the chance for wound infection. Ascher *et al.* [14] have demonstrated that nerve endings cut by the CO₂ laser are sealed rather than left frayed, as by scalpel surgery. This may account for the decreased postoperative pain noted by many after laser surgery.

The minimal damage to adjacent tissue may result in decreased scar formation since dermal elements are minimally damaged. This is in contrast to the excessive scars occurring after electrosurgical injury. However, it may also account for the slightly prolonged healing time after laser surgery. Another benefit from this same factor would be the ability to primarily close a wound with flap or graft immediately after laser surgery since the tissue necrosis debris of electrosurgery is not present.

Having discussed the factors associated with the CO_2 laser as it is used in skin surgery, we may now briefly discuss the various applications to which this laser has been put. Many additional applications will undoubtedly be developed in the future.

Excision of skin lesions

The laser provides a 'light scalpel' with which to excise benign or malignant lesions. This is performed in the focused mode with high-power density. The energy is delivery in a continuous fashion and the depth of the cut is determined inversely by the speed at which the beam is drawn along the target surface. Likewise, the amount of hemostasis is related inversely to the speed of the cut. The articulated arm–handpiece allows the surgeon, with some practice, to perform excisions with the ease of scalpel surgery (Figures 1a and b).

Undermining of wounds can be accomplished by tilting the handpiece or more easily by using an angled mirror tip that deflects the cutting beam at a 90° or 120° angle from the handpiece axis. Such undermining is fast and virtually bloodless. This allows flaps to be cut and mobilized easily with little worry about postoperative hematoma formation (Figures 1c and d). Likewise, grafts can be cut and harvested with the laser and are very viable. The open wound bed after laser excision is very dry and sterile and ready for immediate graft placement.

Mohs' surgery

We have described the CO_2 laser modification of Mohs' surgery [15]. The laser virtually replaces the use of the zinc chloride fixative paste by permitting the bloodless excision of skin cancer with lymphatic closure. Most importantly, the laser preserves perfectly the histology of the cut skin margins so that microscopic control may be achieved. There is no thermal necrosis, as from electrosurgical cutting devices, to distort histology (Figures 2 and 3). The precise cutting of the laser scalpel allows the surgeon to strip away very thin layers of tissue where required. With local anesthesia the procedure is fast and painless and postoperative pain is minimal. Inflammation is avoided, and repair may be performed immediately after completion of the tumor excision. Healing by granulation yields satisfactory scar formation, but may be slightly delayed (Figure 4).

The laser allows the Mohs' surgeon to continue excision into bone if required. At higher-power densities the laser beam is capable of excising thin layers of bone for examination. Equally important is the role of the laser in

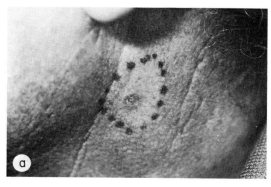

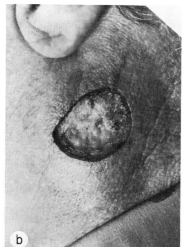

Figure 1 (*a*) Basal cell carcinoma of neck. (*b*) Wound after CO$_2$ laser excision. (*c*) Rotation flap cut and undermined by laser. (*d*) Healing at 3 months

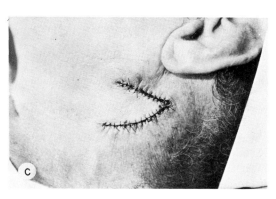

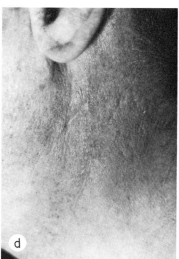

dealing with the problem of exposed raw bone after completion of surgery. This exposed bone usually will take months to be covered with granulation or may not cover at all. The laser is able, at lower-power densities, to vaporize small holes in the bone, exposing the blood supply within. The creation of a vascular grid is accomplished, which speeds granulation and subsequent healing (Figure 5).

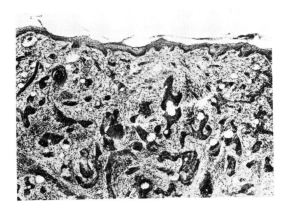

Figure 2   Frozen section of tissue cut by CO_2 laser. Architecture preserved

Figure 3   Frozen section of tissue cut by electrosurgical apparatus. Architecture distorted by thermal necrosis

Tattoo removal

We have described removal of decorative tattoos with the CO_2 laser [16]. This topic is also covered in Chapter 19. It is only necessary to comment that this approach to tattoo removal offers the advantages of being a totally visually controlled, one-step procedure with total pigment ablation. Operative and postoperative discomfort is minimal. It is too early to know whether scar formation following CO_2 laser vaporization is more acceptable than after conventional procedures such as dermabrasion, salabrasion, excision, etc.

Angiokeratomas, cherry hemangiomas, pyogenic granulomas

These small elevated vascular benign tumors are quite amenable to vaporiza-

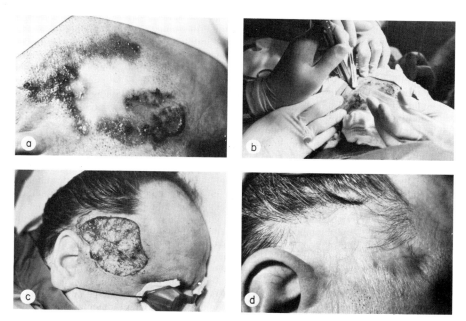

Figure 4 (*a*) Basal cell carcinoma of temple. (*b*) CO_2 laser excision in progress. (*c*) Dry sterile wound immediately postoperatively. (*d*) Healing by granulation. Excellent appearance at 6 months

tion with the CO_2 laser. Treatment is performed at low to medium-power densities in the defocused mode. Pulses of short duration (0.05–0.1 sec) can be used repetitively, or the continuous beam may be brushed back and forth rapidly, in a sense 'erasing' the tumor. Bleeding is minimal to absent. Treatment is stopped (Figure 6) when the skin surface is reached. If a larger feeding vessel is encountered at the base, it may be grasped with forceps or mosquito clamp and the end sealed with the defocused beam.

Lymphangioma circumscriptum

This benign tumor of ectatic lymphatic vessels presents as clustered papules and nodules of cystic character. The channels contain watery colorless lymphatic fluid, and on occasion blood is intermixed. Conventional therapy is by excision or desiccation and curettage. Both are plagued by frequent recurrence.

The CO_2 laser has been used on a few cases of lymphangioma circumscriptum. Vaporization (defocused) is performed with lower-power density and repeated short pulses. The elevated lesions are reduced down to the level of

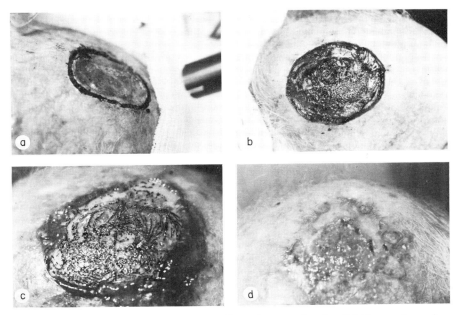

Figure 5   (*a*) CO$_2$ laser excising basal cell carcinoma of scalp. (*b*) Exposed cranium vaporized postoperatively. (*c*) Granulation tissue present on bone at fourth week. (*d*) Entire exposed bone covered by eighth postoperative week

surrounding normal skin. No attempt is made to treat deeper lymphatic structures.

Thus far, results have been excellent with minimal scarring and resolution of the lesions without local recurrence (Figure 7).

Keloids

These tumors of fibrous tissue present a tremendous challenge to the dermatologic surgeon. Excision is usually followed by recurrence, and the adjunctive use of steroid, pressure, and x-ray are only sometimes helpful.

We have used the CO$_2$ laser to excise keloids of earlobes, trunk, and extremities. The keloid is infiltrated with local anesthesia and then shave excised with the laser in a continuous focused mode at high-power density (Figure 8*a–c*). Any remaining fibrotic areas at the wound base or margins are further excised. No closure is performed, nor are any sutures placed. All this is intended to avoid stimulating further fibroplasia. Adjunctively, triamcinolone acetonide 20–40 mg/ml as been injected into the wound base and borders (Figure 8*d*). Wounds have healed in 2–4 weeks with some hypertrophic scarring, but no keloid recurrence (Figure 8*e*).

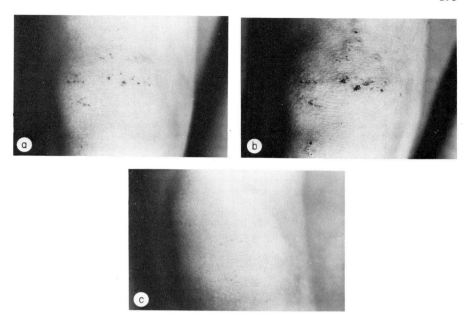

Figure 6   (*a*) Angiokeratomas on knee. (*b*) Immediately after CO$_2$ laser vaporization. (*c*) Three months after treatment

Warts and condylomata acuminata

These viral-induced epithelial tumors are annoying to treat with any modality. Resistance to therapy is common, and recurrences are frequent. Milder, more conservative chemical therapy often requires weeks or months and is often unsuccessful. More aggressive therapy (e.g. desiccation and curettage) may result in significant morbidity, tissue damage, and scarring. Plantar warts and condylomata acuminata are particularly problematic. The CO$_2$ laser is an excellent modality for treating problematic or recurrent warts. In our experience it has now become the method of choice for plantar warts and condylomata acuminata.

The lesions are treated with the laser in a defocused mode at low to medium-power density in a series of brief pulses (0.05–0.1 sec). Treatment is carried out under magnified vision (2.5 × magnifying loupes) in order to see all small satellite warts and to judge more precisely when all wart tissue has been vaporized. Any tissue char is then cleansed away with hydrogen peroxide and the wound base and edges are gently explored with a dull currette. If any residual pockets of wart are discovered, they are vaporized. If no wart remains, the base and edges are lightly vaporized (low-power density) once to sterilize

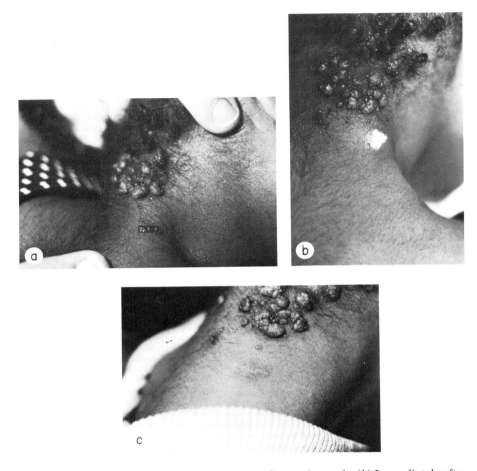

Figure 7   (a) Lymphangioma circumscriptum of posterior neck. (b) Immediately after CO$_2$ laser vaporization of a test area. (c) Excellent healing at 6 months. Scar is flat, supple, slightly hypopigmented

the surface and assure hemostasis. Healing is by granulation and the wounds, even plantar and anogenital, are relatively painless. Healing results in either no scar or a supple flexible scar which is asymptomatic.

This procedure is bloodless and able to be totally visually monitored. The laser beam sterilizes as it destroys, possibly reducing the chance of seeding viral particles and resultant recurrences. Furthermore, the excellent healing and tissue preservation makes treatment on the sole, in the urethral meatus, and vaginal area easier and uncomplicated.

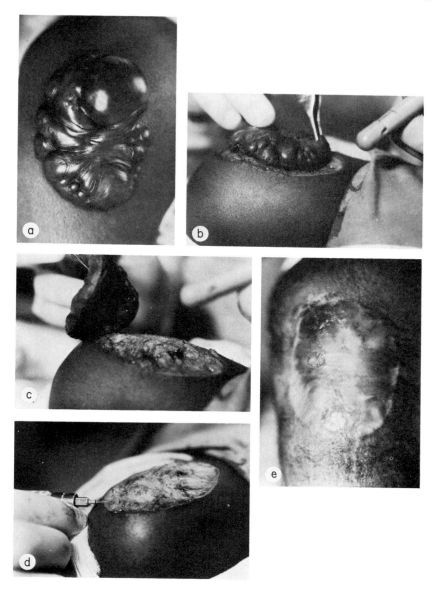

Figure 8 (*a*) Keloid on deltoid area. (*b*) Shave excision with CO$_2$ laser. (*c*) Keloid elevated bloodlessly from base. (*d*) Immediate postoperative injection of wound base with steroid. (*e*) Healed wound at 6 months shows irregular pigment without recurrence of keloid

Epidermal nevi

These developmental defects usually occur on the extremities. They may be removed by excision (single or staged), cryosurgery, or dermabrasion. They often heal with unsatisfactory scarring and tend to recur. The CO_2 laser may be used to rapidly reduce such lesions. With a medium-power density and the beam defocused, the laser is used in the continuous setting. The surgeon sweeps rapidly over the lesion, in effect brushing it away down to the level of surrounding skin. Healing is by granulation and re-epithelialization. The wounds are clean and nonpainful. To help prevent recurrence, treatment with keratolytics (e.g. salicylic acid, lactic acid, etc.) is begun when re-epithelialization is complete.

Summary

The CO_2 laser thus has numerous applications in dermatology and dermatoloic surgery. It is versatile, being either a vaporizing tool or a light scalpel. It produces a dry, sterile operative field which heals beautifully either by immediate closure (flaps, grafts, etc.) or by secondary healing. The post operative period is relatively painless for the patient. Conservation of adjacent tissues is maximized, since thermal energy transfer is minimized.

References

1. McBurney, E. I. Carbon dioxide laser treatment of dermatologic lesions. *South. Med. J.* 1978; **71**:795–7.
2. Kitzmiller, K. W. Laser treatment of tattoos and angiomas. *J. Med. Assoc. Ga.* 1970; **59**:385–6.
3. Goldman, L. Effects of new laser systems on the skin. *Arch. Dermatol.* 1973; **108**:385–90.
4. Goldman, L., Naprstek, Z., Johnson, J. Laser surgery of a digital angiosarcoma: report of a case and six-year follow-up study. *Cancer.* 1977; **39**:1738–42.
5. Olsen, T. G., Milroy, S. K., Goldman, L., *et al.* Laser surgery for blue rubber bleb nevus. *Arch. Dermatol.* 1979; **115**:81–2.
6. Reid, R., Miller, S. Tattoo removal by CO_2 laser dermabrasion. *Plast. Reconstr. Surg.* 1980; **65**:717–28.
7. Klein, D. R. The use of the carbon dioxide laser in plastic surgery. *South. Med. J.* 1977; **70**:429–31.
8. Kaplan, I., Raif, J. The Sharplan carbon dioxide laser in clinical surgery: seven years' experience. In: Goldman, L., ed. *The Biomedical Laser*. New York: Springer-Verlag, 1981:89–98.
9. Schellhas, H. F. Laser surgery in gynecology. In: Goldman, L., ed. *The Biomedical Laser*. New York: Springer-Verlag, 1981:99–106.
10. Landers, M. B., Wolbarsht, M. L. Laser eye instrumentation: diagnostic and surgical. In: Goldman, L., ed. *The Biomedical Laser*. New York: Springer-Verlag, 1981:117–34.

11. Ascher, P. W., Heppner, F. Neurosurgical laser techniques. In: Goldman, L., ed. *The Biomedical Laser*. New York: Springer-Verlag, 1981:219–28.
12. Aronoff, B. L. The carbon dioxide laser in head and neck and plastic surgery: advantages and disadvantages. In: Goldman, L., ed. *The Biomedical Laser*. New York: Springer-Verlag, 1981:239–54.
13. Ben-Bassat, M., Ben-Bassat, M., Kaplan, I. An ultrastructural study of the cut edges of skin and mucous membrane specimens excised by carbon dioxide laser. In: Kaplan I., ed. *Laser Surgery*. Jerusalem: Academic Press, 1976:95–100.
14. Ascher, P., Ingolitsch, E., Walter, G., *et al*. Ultrastructural findings in CNS tissue with CO$_2$ laser. In: Kaplan, I., ed. *Laser Surgery*. Jerusalem: Academic Press, 1976:81–5.
15. Bailin, P. L., Ratz, J. R., Lutz-Nagey, L. CO$_2$ laser modification of Mohs' surgery. *J. Dermatol. Surg. Oncol.* 1981; 7:621–3.
16. Bailin, P. L., Ratz, J. R., Levine, H. L. Removal of tattoos by CO$_2$ laser. *J. Dermatol. Surg. Oncol.* 1980; **6**:997–1001.

Cutaneous Laser therapy: Principles and Methods
Edited by K. A. Arndt, J. M. Noe, and S. Rosen
© 1983 John Wiley & Sons Ltd

19

Laser Treatment of Decorative Tattoos

John A. Dixon

After a period of decreasing popularity, it appears that decorative tattoos are once again being performed with increasing frequency [1]. An American public accustomed to 'impulse buying' is finding that obtaining a tattoo is a relatively permanent decision from which withdrawal is difficult. Previous methods of treatment such as mechanical dermabrasion, salt abrasion, cryosurgery, excision with skin graft, and chemical cauterization all have been effective to some degree, but each is also associated with significant disadvantages such as partial or incomplete removal of pigment, imprecise depth of destruction of tissue, infection, pain, scarring, and the necessity for multiple repeated procedures [2].

The argon and the carbon dioxide laser have both been proposed as modalities for treatment of decorative tattoos [3,4]. This presentation will discuss the technical aspects of laser treatment of tattoos, the results of such treatment, as well as some aspects of scarring, infection, and postoperative wound management.

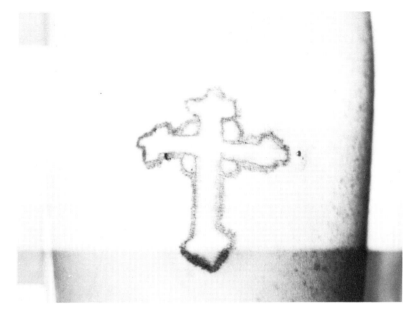

Figure 1   Typical amateur tattoo with India ink. Fuzzy, irregular outlines. Simple
design. Irregular color and depth of pigment

For therapeutic purposes, decorative tattoos may be divided into two categories—amateur and professional. The amateur tattoo, such as that seen in Figure 1, is usually performed by the patient or a friend with a sharp needle using India ink, cigarette ash, shoe polish, pencil lead, charcoal, or other such substance as the pigment. Such tattoos are generally of rather simple design, use a single color, and have irregular blurred outlines. Amateur tattoos are characterized by marked variability in depth of pigment deposition because an inexperienced operator may introduce the pigment into the epidermis, the dermis, or even into subcutaneous fat.

Professional tattoos, such as seen in Figure 2, are accomplished by introducing a broad range of natural chemical compounds chosen for the desired color, such as blue from cobalt, green from chromium, red from mercury, and violet from cobalt and magnesium. The pigment is introduced by a mechanical needle device that embeds the pigment at a generally uniform, relatively superficial depth into the dermis [3]. Such tattoos are usually rather detailed, multicolored, and repesent sharp margins.

The reason depth of pigment deposition is so important in the treatment of tattoos is that the operator must have some concept of the depth of the skin to which one must go to remove the pigment. Although some selective absorption

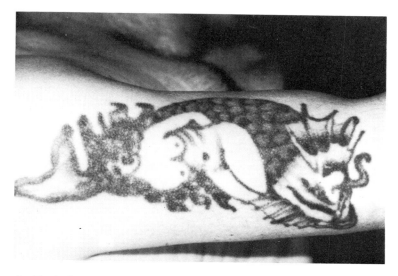

Figure 2 Typical professional tattoo. Sharp margins. Complex design. Even texture and depth of pigment

does take place with certain colored pigments, the laser is really being used in a rather general fashion to plane away the overlying skin so as to physically remove the pigment or to open up the tissues to a point that the pigment is extruded in the post laser therapy period. Even in professional tattoos the depth of deposition of pigment may extend from the basal layer of the epidermis into the papillary and even reticular dermis. The laser treatment must penetrate this level to remove pigment.

The basic steps prior to the application of the laser for treatment of tattoos are essentially the same as those listed for port wine stains (PWS) (see Chapter 11). Again, a careful pretreatment interview is vital in order to review with the patient all aspects of the laser treatments of tattoos with a special emphasis on the probability of white, flat scarring following treatment. Careful inquiry with regard to any previous hypertrophic scarring or keloid formation following injury to the patient is helpful in eliminating treatment to the patient with this type of problem. It is useful to show pre-and postlaser therapy pictures of patients who have had tattoos removed with the argon laser to demonstrate the type of white, flat scarring that has occurred. As might be expected, pain following treatment is considerably more of a problem with these patients than for those with PWS. Analgesics are frequently necessary to provide relief. Excessive pain should prompt a thorough search for localized abscess formation or invasive infection.

Table 1   Technique for treatment of tattoos

(1)	Initial removal of epidermis
(2)	Wipe with hydrogen peroxide
(3)	Initial 1-mm carbonization
(4)	Wipe with hydrogen peroxide
(5)	Second 1-mm carbonization
(6)	Wipe
(7)	If necessary, third 1-mm carbonization
(8)	Wipe
(9)	Spot treat any small areas of remaining pigment

Technique (Table 1)

Argon laser treatment

Anesthesia is obtained in most of these patients by local infiltration of an agent such as 4 percent prilocaine. The local anesthetic is injected intradermally through a 30-gauge flexible needle. Only that portion of the tattoo that can be removed in 20–30 min is infiltrated at one time so as to preclude loss of anesthetic effect and necessity for reinjection and hence introduction of more of the anesthetic agent. In large tattoos, care should be taken not to exceed the recommended maximal dose per kilogram of that agent for a given patient, inasmuch as these lesions are very large and considerable amounts of anesthetic agent are required. The area of a tattoo that can be handled under local anesthesia usually coincides well with the amount the patient can tolerate at one given time. This area generally can be up to a maximum of 12 square inches.

Complete removal of the epidermis and some of the dermis is required to remove the pigment, and therefore care must be exercised to avoid introducing bacteria into the wound. A 'clean' technique is utilized, recognizing that a sterile technique is almost impossible in these circumstances. The skin is washed with pHisohex, sterile gloves are worn, the laser fiber is wiped off with alcohol prior to use by the operator.

The argon laser may be applied by an intermittent technique or by a continuous technique. In either case, the power setting should be sufficient to produce whitening, wrinkling, and vesiculation of the epidermis with the initial pass and carbonization with subsequent applications. In the intermittent technique, settings of 1.8–2.5 W, 2-mm spot size, with duration of application of 0.2–0.4 sec are usually required. With the continuous technique, settings are usually 1.8–2.5 W and the rapidity of passage over the skin is judged by tissue reaction. These settings generally result in skin irradiance of 30–60 J/cm^2.

The technique used is similar to that described by Bailin *et al.* [4]. The initial pass of the laser is designed to remove all of the epidermis and expose the underlying dermis with its embedded pigment to more intense laser power densities. The entire lesion is treated to the point where the superficial skin is white, wrinkled, and vesicular, and can be easily wiped off. The treatment should extend at least 2 mm beyond the margins of any visible pigment, as a common cause for retreatment is pigment deposition extending slightly outside the margins of the treated area. In tattoos involving figures or letters with small islands of normal skin, the normal skin is included in the treatment. Initially, this normal skin was allowed to remain and resulted in irregular contour of the treated area with a 'ghost' appearance of the now nonpigmented design; this was very distressing to the patient. By converting a definitive outline to an ambiguous uniform area, the appearance of a purposefully created lesion is dispelled.

Following this initial treatment, the superficially photocoagulated layer is wiped off using a surgical sponge soaked in hydrogen peroxide contained in a sterile basin. The treated area should be rubbed vigorously with a sponge. The treated skin wipes off readily. The operator is almost always amazed at the very intense, vivid colors that appear as the pigmented dermis is then exposed following removal of the epidermis.

The next step consists of an intense application of the laser over all pigmented areas thus exposed. This should create a charred appearance extending to a depth of approximately 1 mm. Small islands of normal skin are likewise treated to this depth. The margins of the tattoo are beveled so as to avoid a shelf appearance. At the conclusion of this application, it will look like the entire tattoo has been removed and the skin carbonized deeply.

Once again, the hydrogen peroxide-soaked sponge is rubbed vigorously over the treated area. On all but the most superficial tattoos, the operator will be once again amazed to see the carbon wipe off along with a great deal of pigment, and the color and outline of the tattoo clearly reappear. A second deep application of the laser is then carried out exactly as previously described.

The lesion is again wiped vigorously with hydrogen peroxide. At this point the outline of the tattoo may appear indistinct with only a small amount of pigment remaining. If this is the case the treatment may be concluded. If not, one more application (just the same as previously described) is carried out and the lesion again wiped. It has been our practice not to exceed three general applications of the laser to the tattooed area because of depth of penetration. If small amounts of pigment are remaining in small spots, these may be removed on the fourth round but no general treatment is carried out. A summary of these applications appears in Figure 3. At this time nearly all the pigment should have been removed. It is not uncommon to have a faint general outline of the lesion remaining due to small amounts of carbon remaining in the pigmented area or even some remaining pigment. This will generally be

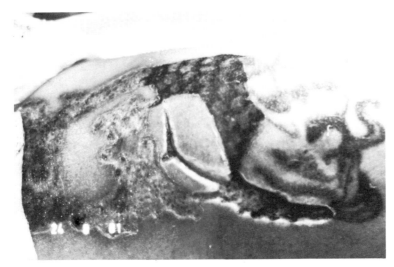

Figure 3   Stages of tattoo removal. From bottom of figure to top: pretreatment; following first pass—epidermis removal; following third pass—deep carbonization; 10 days post-treatment healing

extruded but can be further removed with a small curette if desired. Experience with fourth and even fifth applications resulted in prolonged healing and greater thickening of resulting scar. In those patients in whom it appears some deeper pigment is embedded, it is preferable to advise them that the pigment was very deeply embedded and may require areas of touch-up following healing. It is not unusual to see a few small areas of remaining pigment that require subsequent removal, even in the more superficial lesions. This usually requires little time and is well tolerated by the patient. Figure 3 illustrates stages of pretreatment, superficial epidermis removal, carbonization, and healing in the same tattoo.

A thin film of bacitracin ointment is then applied to the treated area and a sterile nonocclusive gauze dressing applied. The postoperative wound care is very similar to that described in Chapter 11 for PWS, although frequent dressing is required for a longer period of time. Mild analgesics such as provided by codeine derivative are frequently required.

It is useful to very carefully describe to the patient what might be expected with the healing sequence of the wound. Initially, there will be the formation of a brownish crust. The patient may shower or sponge the area but should not cause maceration by excessive soaking with water or excessive application of ointment. These crusts will remain from 2 to 4 weeks depending upon the depth of the treatment. Following slough of the crust, the lesion will appear flat, indented, shiny, and very pink to purple due to the reaction of healing. Patients are instructed that it will be at least 9 months to a year before healing is complete. Any remaining pigment may be removed at any time following 3 months of healing.

Because of the depth and extent of these lesions, invasive infection has been seen in two of 30 patients. This is usually heralded by increased pain and discharge in the area of the wound, plus lymphangitis, cellulitis, chills and fever. Following culture, appropriate antibiotics are administered which usually control this complication in 2–3 days.

Because of the depth of vaporization necessary to remove the pigment, nearly all of these patients will have a scar which consists of a white, flat, lattice-like reaction. Surprisingly, thick, hypertrophic scars have been rare. If such scars are noted, they can be treated in the same fashion as outlined in the paragraphs on scarring in Chapter 11. Jobst pressure dressings are particularly applicable on these lesions of the extremities.

Carbon dioxide (CO₂) laser treatment

As described by Bailin et al.[4], tattoos may be effectively removed utilizing the CO_2 laser and the exact same 'wipe' technique as just described for the argon laser. Although some selective absorption is noted with the argon laser, the basic modality with both lasers appears to be 'planing away' the epidermis and dermis to the level at which the pigment is either removed or allowed to extrude. We have noted similar results in our patients with either CO_2 or argon laser treatment. In four patients, half of a tattoo was treated with the CO_2 and half with the argon laser. There were no discernible differences between the treated halves and such result is illustrated in Figure 4. The patients reported that the CO_2-treated lesions were somewhat more painful postoperatively.

The general range of settings for CO_2 treatments is 6–8 W, continuous power for removal of the epidermis, and deeper dermal vaporization using the articulating arm. Using the intermittent spot technique, similar results can be obtained by using 6–8 W at 0.2 sec. The operating microscope attachment may be used, but is more tedious and time consuming.

Results

Utilizing this technique, the results of tattoo removal on 30 patients followed for more than one year at the University of Utah were determined by physician evaluation as follows:

Number of patients	30
Average number of treatments	2.4
Excellent result	0
Good result	97 percent
Poor result	3 percent
Hypertrophic scar	7 percent

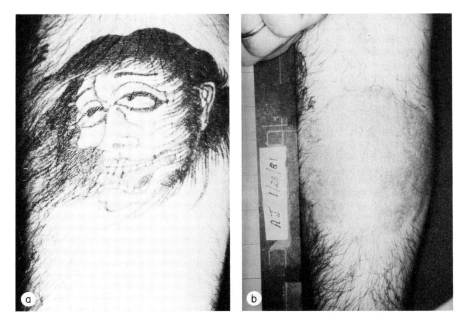

Figure 4 (*a*) Control argon/CO_2 comparison tattoo, pretreatment. (*b*) Comparison tattoo, upper half argon treated, lower half CO_2 treated. No discernible difference

Eighty-seven percent of these patients reported overall satisfaction with the results of their laser treatment (R. H. Rotering, personal communication). These results are roughly comparable to those in the series reported by Apfelberg *et al.* [1]. Good removal of pigment was obtained in nearly all patients. Excellent results were not recorded because of the white, flat scars. Despite the irregular, whitish appearance following healing, these patients are generally very grateful to be relieved of the pigmented tattoo and all the surrounding memories and sequelae.

Typical good results are seen in Figure 5. Subsequent 'filling-in' and more normal pigmentation may occur up to 18 months post-treatment. Several small remaining islands of skin would have been removed in the more recent technique described.

Discussion

Inasmuch as it is necessary to remove pigment in the papillary and reticular dermis, some postoperative scarring is almost inevitable. It is of great importance to evaluate the patient carefully prior to treatment for any tendency toward keloid formation. Examination of previous incisions, lacerations, or vaccination scars is useful in identifying excessive tendency to

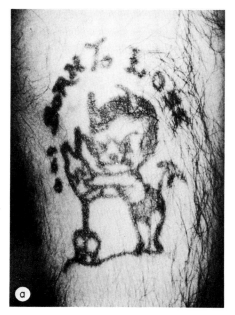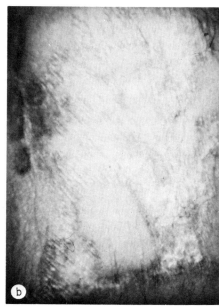

Figure 5 (*a*) Professional tattoo, pretreatment. (*b*) One year post-treatment. Good pigment removal. White scar shows some 'skin islands'. No keloid

scar formation. Nearly all but the most superficial tattoos will demonstrate a very fine, white, flat latticework of scar deposition. This is generally considered to be acceptable by the patient and is viewed as a considerable improvement over the tattoo. Thickened ropelike scars occur in 7–10 percent of patients. These are particularly likely to appear in treatments over the deltoid, exterior thoracic, and flexor and extensor creases. Very large or long linear tattoos usually predispose to heavier scar formation. Hypertrophic scars are treated by the injection of intralesional triamcinolone acetonide (Kenalog, 40 mg/ml) and Cordran tape.

Initially, only the pigmented areas of tattoos were removed. It was soon evident that in a number of cases an indented, whitish 'ghost' with islands of normal skin had been substituted for what had been the original tattoo. In tattoos involving numbers, letters, and single-line drawings, the outline of the tattoo was almost as evident as in its prior pigmented state. At the present this is avoided by circumscribing the entire tattoo with a line such that the resultant figure will be indeterminate, ambiguous, and not recognizable as any particular form, letter, or number. Within the outline, nonpigmented normal skin areas will be treated as well as pigmented ones. The unpigmented skin is treated only slightly less deeply than is the pigmented, so as to avoid leaving unsightly islands of normal skin in the center of the tattoo. The external line is carefully made with the laser so as to be slightly outside any pigmented portion of the tattoo. One of the most frequent reasons for retreatment has been the failure to treat at least 1 mm outside the margin of any evident pigment. This mistake results in a spotty peripheral outline of the former tattoo.

It is, of course, entirely possible to assure complete removal of all pigment at the first treatment. Such assurance is obtained at the expense of more pain, prolonged healing, increased scarring, and potential third-degree burn. Present practice is to be conservative on depth of initial vaporization and to inform patients that a touch-up will likely be necessary.

Infection will occur in nearly all of these lesions following treatment. It is usually very superficial, noninvasive, and controlled by the topical antibiotic ointment. In three patients it was necessary to give systemic antibiotics for cellulitis and lymphangitis in the region of the treated area.

The personality and behavior of these patients is interesting. A group of them are professional people, actors, TV personalities, clergymen, and housewives. These individuals are usually of the 'it was a great party; it seemed like a good idea at the time; I was surprised when it wouldn't wash off the next morning' variety. The other group is a strange mixture in whom the tattoo has been incurred in association factors such as with a gang, prison, armed forces, subculture, social beliefs, harsh raising in an institution, organized crime, or sexual preference. The second group is further characterized by failure to keep appointments, failure to follow postoperative instructions, failure to return for evaluation, and, naturally, failure to pay their bills. A rather unique observation in this group was that several of them complained of extreme pain postopertively, requiring patient-specified narcotics for relief. Contacts with local law enforcement officers disclosed that several of these patients had financed their tattoo removal by street sale of narcotics obtained during the postoperative period by such complaints of pain.

Summary

In summary, the treatment of decorative tattoos with argon or CO_2 lasers is a distinct advance over previous techniques and is associated with a high degree of patient satisfaction. In order to remove all pigment, especially in amateur tattoos, a vigorous sequential operative removal of pigment is essential. One later retreatment is frequently necessry to remove small residues. White, flat, 'acceptable' scarring occurs in nearly all patients. Three percent of patients may have some hypertrophic scarring. Tattooed patients from some societal elements have difficulty carrying through a treatment program. The treatment is time consuming, painful, and not without some risk due to infection. Patients generally are gratified and pleased with their final result in a high percentage of cases.

References

1. Apfelberg, D. B., Maser, M. R., Lash, H. Argon laser treatment of decorative tattoos. *Br. J. Plast. Surg.* 1979; **32**:141–4.
2. Boa-Chai, K. The decorative tattoo: its removal by dermabrasion. *Plast. Reconstr. Surg.* 1963; **32**:559–68.
3. Apfelberg, D. B., Taub, D. R., Maser, M. R., *et al.* Pathophysiology and treatment of decorative tattoos with reference to argon laser treatment. *Clin. Plast. Surg.* 1980; **7**:369–77.
4. Bailin, P. L., Ratz, J. L., Levine, H. L. Removal of tattoos by CO_2 laser. *J. Dermatol. Surg. Oncol.* 1980; **6**:997–1001.

Psychosocial Aspects of Facial Disfigurement and the Effects of Modification via Laser Therapy

Cutaneous Laser Therapy: Principles and Methods
Edited by K. A. Arndt, J. M. Noe, and S. Rosen
© 1983 John Wiley & Sons Ltd

20

Laser Treatment of Port Wine Stains: Observations Concerning Psychological Outcome

S. Michael Kalick

There is much reason to believe that the patient who seeks laser treatment for a port wine stain (PWS) wishes to alleviate not just a physical ailment but also an important source of psychological stress. Therefore, it is most useful for physicians who treat these patients to have an awareness of the psychological and social consequences of a PWS as well as its physical chracteristics. In a recent article, Kalick, Goldwyn, and Noe [1] presented research findings concerning PWS patients' life experiences and the social forces that help account for them, as well as their perceptions and reactions to a laser clinic as they began the process of treatment. This presentation follows the same patient

Table 1   Laser psychosocial monitoring program

Stage of treatment	Stage of monitoring
Initial interview with surgeon completed	(1) Psychosocial survey (2) Standard personality tests
Test patch completed	First psychosocial follow-up
First treatment completed	Second psychosocial follow-up
Second treatment completed	Third psychosocial follow-up
Final treatment completed	(1) Postcompletion follow-up (2) Standard personality tests readministered
Approximately 18 months after final treatment (*or* after dropping out)	Long-term follow-up (*or* long-term dropout follow-up)

sample through the completion of treatment and two years beyond. The aim here is to discuss the psychological factors initially deemed important for understanding PWS patients and to shed light on other factors that appear to be related to patient satisfaction or dissatisfaction with the results of treatment.

It is worthwhile at the outset to review and amplify the sampling and survey the methodology used in this research. The patients were among the first to be treated for PWS lesions at the argon laser facility located at Boston's Beth Israel Hospital. Patients in this sample began treatment at approximately the start of 1978. Efforts were made at coordinating investigation at the laser facility among the disciplines of plastic surgery, dermatology, pathology, psychology, and nursing care [1–4]. This later research is based substantially, although not entirely, on the same group of patients.

Each patient's regimen began with a consultation with the plastic surgeon, followed by a 'test patch' laser treatment in a small, relatively inconspicuous area of the PWS to help determine whether or not to proceed. For those patients with encouraging test patch results, the PWS was treated in segments. This generally involved several treatment sessions, spaced approximately 3 months apart. The time sequence has proved to be appropriate for a long-term psychosocial investigation.

As shown in Table 1, patients were asked to supply information at six points in time before, during, and after their treatment. At each of these points the patients were given specially prepared psychosocial survey forms to fill out and return. The survey materials concentrated at first on exploring the personal consequences of having lived with a PWS and the anticipated consequences of laser treatment. Subsequent surveys focused on the actual experience of going through the treatment program. The final two survey forms dealt mainly with the patients' estimates of the laser program and its effects on their lives, their expectations of the future, advice to prospective laser patients, and in general what they had learned from their experience. The complete set of survey materials comprised some 20 pages per patient and included a number of scales on which the patient had to circle a number, as well as numerous open-ended questions that offered an opportunity to respond in depth.

Patients also responded to a set of standardized psychological tests, chosen because they measure traits considered important for understanding the PWS patient. The test instruments included the Eysenck Personality Inventory [5], the Multiple Affect Adjective Checklist [6], the Spielberger Self-Report Inventory [7], and the Coopersmith Self-Report Form [8]. Table 2 specifies the characteristics measured by each of the tests; these include the degree of outgoing personality, neurotic personality, depression, hostility, self-esteem, and several categories of anxiety. As shown in Table 1, the psychological tests were administered in conjunction with the pretreatment survey forms, and were readministered in conjunction with the postcompletion survey materials. These two points in time were almost always at least one year apart.

The multidisciplinary research sample consisted of 100 patients who began treatment during the first few months of the laser clinic's operation. These patients were asked to participate in the psychosocial research, and 82 consented and returned the initial monitoring materials. After the test patch session, 80 patients continued their participation in our research by returning the first psychosocial follow-up. By the second follow-up—after the first full-scale treatment—the sample diminished to 57 patients. The third follow-up comprised data from 33 patients, and the post completion materials were returned by 29 patients. This attrition is not unexpected in research carried out over a long period of time. The postcompletion follow-up figure of 29 patients, in fact, corresponds closely to the proportion of the initial 82 who actually received a 'final' treatment. About 60 percent of the initial sample did not reach this event; some discontinued in response to an unencouraging result of the test patch or first treatment, others moved away or otherwise lost touch with us, others travel to the clinic very sporadically and are still in the process of treatment, while yet others have suspended treatment and are awaiting improvements in the laser modality.

The attrition is a cause for methodologic concern in that it may have brought about many differences in aggregate characteristics between the pretreatment and postcompletion samples. Such comparisons thus involve some hazard since they may tap attrition effects rather than treatment effects. This issue has been handled in two ways. First, whenever two or more points in time are compared, only those patients are included who provided information at each of the relevant times. Second, a long-term follow-up survey was carried out, as shown in Table 1, and both completion patients and dropout patients responded. As will be detailed below, the inclusion of dropout data as well as completion data in several instances improved our ability to draw valid and clear-cut conclusions.

Table 2   The psychological test instruments

Name of test	Characteristic measured
Eysenck Personality Inventory	(1) Extroversion vs introversion (2) Neurotic personality
Multiple Affect Adjective Checklist	(1) Anxiety (2) Depression (3) Hostility
Spielberger Self-Report Inventory	(1) Anxiety as (transient) state (2) Anxiety as a character trait
Coopersmith Self-Report Form	Self-esteem

Table 3   Pearson correlations between severity of PWS and psychological test scores

	Correlation $(r)^*$
Severity with:	
Extroversion	0.01
Neurotic personality	0.08
Anxiety ('MAACL')	0.07
Depression	0.08
Hostility	0.07
Transient anxiety	0.01
Anxiety as a trait	0.03
Self-esteem	0.12

$^*r$ signifies Pearson produce–moment correlation.

Psychological characteristics of PWS patients

As discussed in detail by Kalick *et al.* [1], the pretreatment battery of psychological tests failed to find noteworthy differences between the patient sample, taken as an aggregate, and the 'normal' comparison groups whose data were supplied by the test makers. The relative normality of the PWS patient sample is in contrast to a high incidence of psychological disturbance found among a variety of cosmetic plastic surgery patients studied some time ago by Edgerton *et al.* [9] and Reich [10]. However, more recent research carried out by Goin *et al.* [11] with a specific cosmetic surgery population (face-lift patients) showed that their patients presented a relatively normal psychological profile. The finding of relative normality in the aggregate, of course, does not imply that the physician is immune from encountering an occasional deeply disturbed patient who must be handled with caution in the manner, for example, described in the excellent book by Goin and Goin [12].

Aside from aggregate comparison between PWS patients and a control population, there is also the issue of differences among the patients themselves. One question is whether a relatively severe PWS lesion as opposed to a mild one tends to impose a greater psychological burden that can be detected in one or more aspects of character structure. Severity of PWS was available for use as a variable with our patient sample. It was calculated for each patient as a composite measure of the surface area and color of the lesion. Table 3 shows the correlation between lesion severity and each of the pretreatment psychological test scores. The most striking feature of this table is how close to zero all the correlations are. Apparently, the patients are able to cope with even severe PWS lesions in ways that do not bring about personality malformations, at least insofar as the test instruments are able to detect.

Another issue of concern is whether male and female patients present consistent differences in their psychological profiles. Past research has found that male cosmetic-surgery patients tend to be more psychologically disturbed than their female counterparts [12,13]. One plausible explanation for this finding is that appearance-altering surgery has been a relatively 'frowned upon' option for men in our society, so that only quite troubled men would tend to resort to it. This option has perhaps been viewed more leniently for women, thus lowering their threshold for pursuing it and making female patients more representative of women in general. Aside from the fact that cultural standards seem to be becoming increasingly lenient for both sexes, it is not likely that cultural sanctions against males resorting to cosmetic surgery would extend to their seeking treatment for a PWS. Therefore, one would not expect male PWS patients to be notably more psychologically disturbed than females. The pretreatment data, in fact, show no statistically significant sex differences in introversion/extroversion, self-esteem, or any of the categories of anxiety that were measured. The females did score significantly higher on the neurotic personality scale ($t = 2.29$,* $P < 0.05$), while the males scored significantly higher on the depression scale ($t = 2.54$, $P < 0.05$) and higher by an amount that just falls short of statistical significance on the hostility scale ($t = 2.00$, $P < 0.06$). An attempted interpretation of this pattern of differences would be speculative at best at this point; ideally, data from other PWS patient samples should first be sought to see whether the pattern repeats itself. However, these data clearly do not support the simple conclusion that the male patients are more psychologically disturbed than the females.

An additional issue of interest regarding the psychological test instruments is the question of whether they successfully predict who will stay the course of treatment and who will drop out. The converse possibility is that patients drop out of treatment because of nonpsychological factors such as unencouraging early results or geographic mobility. In comparing the completion patients with those who did not complete the program, one finds no statistically significant differences on any of the psychological scales. However, differences approached statistical significance on three of the scales. Noncompletion patients tended to score higher on neuroticism ($t = 1.71$, $P < 0.1$), hostility ($t - 1.87$, $P < 0.1$), and trait anxiety ($t = 1.82$, $P < 0.1$) than completion patients scored on the pretreatment tests. This suggests that psychological factors do play some role in a patient's persisting through the treatment process to completion. This role appears to be relatively minor, though, compared with extrinsic factors. Noncompletion patients, for example, experienced a poorer 'early objective treatment result' (to be discussed in detail below) than completion patients, by a highly significant margin ($t = 4.08$, $P < 0.001$).

Correlates of patient satisfaction with treatment

Patient satisfaction, a peripheral issue with regard to life-saving or life-sustaining procedures, assumes central importance for procedures aimed primarily at improving appearance. With such procedures, a result deemed successful by the physician may be associated with an unfavorable overall outcome if the patient is for some reason dissatisfied. While the complexity of factors underlying patient satisfaction should not be underestimated, the psychosocial monitoring program has provided grounds for at least a preliminary assessment of the bases for satisfaction/dissatisfaction with PWS laser treatment. With the cautionary note that these findings are indeed preliminary, the correlates we have observed can be presented.

Each of the psychosocial follow-up questionnaires asked patients to specify their level of satisfaction with the treatment program. For the sake of uncluttered presentation, we will focus on data from three points in time:

(1) the follow-up subsequent to the first treatment;

(2) the postcompletion follow-up; and

(3) the long-term follow-up (see Table 1).

Where specified, data from the long-term dropout follow-up also will be included. The first treatment follow-up asked patients how successful, on a four-point scale, the laser had been in treating their test patch area. Therefore this item will be referred to as test patch satisfaction. The postcompletion item (and the dropout follow-up item) asked patients to specify, on a six-point scale, how satisfied they were with the laser program and its effects upon their lives. The long-term follow-up item asked patients to specify, on a seven-point scale, their overall satisfaction with the laser treatment program and its effects upon them. Many patients also wrote elaborate in-depth comments, but for present purposes the quantitative data will prove easier to deal with.

Pretreatment personality pattern

The observation presented earlier, that standard personality measures are at most of mild explanatory power for understanding our patient sample, is corroborated when the personality scores are examined in relation to satisfaction with treatment. Table 4 presents the correlations between each of the psychological test scores and self-rated satisfaction at three points in time as specified above. Of the 24 correlations presented in this table, only three achieve statistical significance. Extroversion, although not significantly correlated with test patch satisfaction or postcompletion satisfaction, is significantly related to long-term satisfaction ($r = 0.41$,† $P < 0.05$). Patients higher in pretreatment extroversion tended to register greater satisfaction with

Table 4   Pearson correlations between psychological test scores and satisfaction with treatment

Personality measure	Satisfaction score		
	After test patch $(r)^*$	After final treatment $(r)^*$	Long-term follow-up $(r)^*$
Extroversion	−0.07	0.14	0.41†
Neurotic personality	0.08	−0.21	0.13
Anxiety ('MAACL')	−0.01	−0.29	0.22
Depression	−0.03	−0.35†	0.18
Hostility	−0.12	−0.31	0.28
Transient anxiety	−0.10	−0.15	−0.02
Anxiety as a trait	0.05	−0.26	0.17
Self-esteem	0.00	0.42†	0.22

*r signifies Pearson product–moment correlation.
†$P < 0.05$.

treatment when surveyed 1–2 years after completion. Pretreatment depression was negatively correlated with postcompletion satisfaction ($r = -0.035$, $P < 0.05$). This implies that patients who were more depressed pretreatment tended to be less satisfied after the final treatment. Pretreatment self-esteem was positively correlated with postcompletion satisfaction ($r = 0.42$, $P < 0.05$). Neither of these relationships remained statistically significant by the time of the long-term folow-up, and, indeed, the depression/satisfaction relationship actually reversed direction: patients higher in pretreatment depression tended to be more satisfied when surveyed 1–2 years after completion. At this point it would be venturesome, indeed, to use any psychological measure to predict future patients' satisfaction with laser treatment.

Early objective result

The current state of the art of laser therapy, as discussed elsewhere in this book, does not make it possible to provide all PWS patients with a uniformly excellent treatment result. Patient selection on the basis of likelihood of favorable result is therefore important. Rule-of-thumb criteria, most prominently lesion color, are currently in wide use. The patients discussed here received a small test patch treatment which was evaluated some 4 months later to determine whether the prospects were favorable for successful full-scale treatment. Two components of this 4-month evaluation are combined here to form a measure that will be referred to as 'early objective result'. The two components are: degree of chromatic lightening (the difference between original color and treated color), and physician's overall estimate of whether the result is desirable or undesirable (this is based on scarring and other factors).

Since the patient's evaluation is ultimately far more important than the physician's, it is interesting to see how well early objective result correlates with the patients' satisfaction ratings. In fact, there is a highly significant correlation between early objective result and the patients' test patch satisfaction ($r = 0.05$, $P < 0.001$). However, the correlation between early objective result and postcompletion satisfaction dwindles to an r value of 0.12; this is not statistically significant. The correlation between early objective result and long-term satisfaction gives an r value of 0.18; again, not statistically significant.

These data, at first glance, give cause for serious concern. The physician's early evaluation seems to agree well with the patients' evaluations at the same point in time, but predict poorly indeed who will be satisfied by the end of treatment. Fortunately, the explanation for this finding vindicates the usefulness of early objective result as a predictive measure, at the same time clarifying the limits of its predictive power. It happens that, by the time patients reach the final treatment, those with a relatively poor early objective result tend to have already dropped out—in other words, by this point in time the distribution of this measure has been severely truncated. Its correlation with satisfaction can therefore be expected to decline. Inclusion of data from the dropout follow-up along with data from the completion patients can give a clearer picture of the realationship between early objective result and eventual satisfaction with the treatment program. Once the data are thus pooled, the correlation between early result and long-term satisfaction indeed turns out to be substantial and highly statistically significant ($r = 0.67$, $P < 0.001$).

What can be concluded from this pattern of findings is that the physician's early evaluation provides the basis for an effective screening procedure. It differentiates reasonably well between those patients who ought and those who ought not to proceed (although each physician would have to arrive at his/her precise dividing line). However, among those patients who receive a 'green light', early result provides a weak basis for predicting who will finish with an excellent as opposed to merely a good result.

Severity of lesion

In past psychologically oriented writing, much has been made of the 'cosmetic' patient with minimal disfigurement [12]. This patient has often been assumed to pose a hazard to the practitioner, in that excessive perfectionism and/or psychological disturbance have been held to make this sort of patient

Table 5   Pearson correlations between severity ratings of PWS and satisfaction with treatment

Severity rating	Satisfaction score		
	After test-patch $(r)^*$	After final treatment $(r)^*$	Long-term follow-up $(r)^*$
Composite severity measure	0.02	−0.16	−0.44†
Surface area of lesion	−0.01	−0.23	−0.51†

$^*r$ signifies Pearson produce–moment correlation.
†$P < 0.05$.

unlikely to be satisfied. Severity of lesion has already been shown, as discussed earlier, to be essentially uncorrelated with psychological disturbances, insofar as we could detect, among our sample.

The top row of Table 5 shows the correlations between our composite severity measure and patient satisfaction at three points in time. The two variables prove to be uncorrelated at the outset, but become increasingly negatively correlated over time. By the time of the long-term follow-up, patients who had had more severe original lesions were significantly *less* likely to be satisfied with treatment ($r = 0.44$, $P < 0.05$). The components of our severity measure—lesion color and lesion surface area—were separately examined. It was found, as shown in the bottom row of Table 5, that the entire relationship between severity and satisfaction is accounted for by surface area of lesion (darkness of lesion, in fact, correlates positively with satisfaction). Patients with larger original lesions tended to be less satisfied with the results of treatment, and this tendency grew stronger over time.

It is difficult to interpret this finding with certainty. An educated guess is that larger lesions increase the possibility that some part of the lesion will fade less well than the rest or else sustain some degree of scarring. This possibility would have unfolded only over time, as more and more of the lesion was treated. It seems reasonable to suggest that special care should be taken, in initial consultation, to warn patients with large lesions that their PWS might fade unevenly or sustain scars in places. Also, to the extent that these hazards exist, treatment measures that minimize them will certainly prove to be favorable developments.

Sex of patient

As mentioned earlier, our findings show no consistent pattern of greater psychological disturbance in males as opposed to females or vice versa. This is in contrast with previous writings which suggest special caution with male 'cosmetic' patients. The present data do happen to suggest a relationship between sex of patient and satisfaction with treatment. The females registered significantly higher test patch satisfaction ($t = 2.31$, $P < 0.05$) and postcompletion satisfaction ($t = 2.12$, $P < 0.05$) than the males. By the time of the long-term follow-up, however, the difference disappeared and both sexes averaged the same amount of satisfaction with treatment.

It should be emphasized that even the males, on the whole, were quite satisfied with treatment. In the postcompletion survey, for example, 82 percent of the male respondents indicated at least some degree of satisfaction. However, to the extent that there was any difference between the sexes, it was the females who tended to be somewhat more satisfied.

Unexpected events

Prior to the decision to commence laser treatment, the physician informed all patients in our sample of a number of potential hazards, including the chance of scarring, uneven lightening of the PWS, and the likely temporary manifestations of a local wound. As discussed by Kalick et al. [1], patients often failed either to comprehend or to remember many of the possible events about which the physician had warned them in initial consultation. This raises the sobering possibility of surprise, disappointment, anger, or worse, once treatment is begun.

Since our survey materials ask patients about both unexpected discoveries and satisfaction with treatment, we were able to determine whether unexpected events are, in fact, associated with reduced satisfaction. According to our data, they are not. Patients who reported unexpected happenings, or who reported that the test patch was a more difficult experience than they had expected, did not as a group indicate a significantly lower level of satisfaction than the other patients at any point in our monitoring program. This absence of a significant relationship we attribute to the atmosphere of considerateness and understanding that we try to foster in the laser clinic. Physicians and staff, by being highly supportive toward patients, were perhaps able to compensate for and smooth over the element of surprise on most occasions when it arose. We hope we are not flattering ourselves undeservedly.

Treatment by physician and staff

Considering that the laser clinic is organized around a concrete, physically defined intervention, the importance of interpersonal interactions can easily be underestimated. Our survey materials tapped this aspect of treatment in several ways, but most unambiguously in the following question that patients were aksed: 'How would you rate your satisfaction with the way you were treated by your doctor and the rest of the staff?' A seven-point scale was provided for patients' responses. Our finding is that this measure correlates substantially with test patch satisfaction ($r = 0.34$, $P < 0.1$) as well as postcompletion satisfaction ($r = 0.39$, $P < 0.1$), and it correlates significantly with long-term satisfaction ($r = 0.47$, $P < 0.05$). It will be recalled that the test patch measure asks patients to rate the success of treatment to that point, the postcompletion measure asks for their satisfaction with the treatment's effect on their lives, and the long-term measure asks for overall satisfaction with treatment and its effects on them. It should not escape notice that these three measures are more strongly related to satisfaction with physician and staff than to any of the psychological test scores we discussed earlier.

This finding serves to underline the piece of wisdom offered frequently in the past but perhaps rarely appreciated to the full extent of its worth: medical treatment is far more than an impersonal interaction. The quality of the human interaction plays a large role in determining the meaning of the entire experience for the patient's life, and may well, as a consequence, influence the actual degree of healing that takes place. The crucial patient–clinician interaction has received thoughtful in-depth treatment by two recent authors, Cousins [14] from the standpoint of the patient and Goldwyn [15] from the standpoint of the clinician.

The outcome of laser therapy

It is of perhaps questionable merit to describe the psychological outcome of treatment in global terms, since each patient's individual experience is unique, important, and, at most, vaguely determined by the overall probabilities. However, since an exhaustive compendium of individual experiences is not appropriate here, the most that can be attempted is a faithful rendering of the aggregate.

In considering the possibility that treatment might bring about some changes in personality, we administered the battery of psychological tests before the start of treatment and again along with the postcompletion materials (see Tables 1 and 2). The data permitted a repeated-measures statistical comparison of each pretreatment score with the score on the corresponding psychological scale after treatment was completed. These comparisons yielded no significant differences, nor any marginally significant differences, nor even the hint of a trend. We simply could not detect personality changes that correspond to the completion of laser treatment. This observation is in line with the long-held opinion of Frances C. Macgregor that appearance-altering procedures, particularly in adults, alter not personality but modes of coping within an established personality [16].

Another set of items that was repeated from the pretreatment to the postcompletion survey was a series of specific life-satisfaction measures. Patients were asked to specify their degree of satisfaction with: 'your

Table 6   Patients' evaluations* of various aspects of their life experience before and after laser treatment

Evaluation Rating

Aspect of life experience	Before treatment	After final treatment	Significance of difference
Satisfaction with same-sex relationships	3.69	3.83	NS
Satisfaction with opposite-sex relationships	3.38	3.80	$P < 0.001$
Satisfaction with self as a person	3.34	3.59	NS
Satisfaction with life in general	3.66	3.66	NS

*Based on four-point scale.

relationships with people of the same sex as yourself', 'your relationships with people of the opposite sex', 'yourself as a person', and 'your life in general'. Each of these items was followed by a four-point scale ranging from 'very dissatisfied' to 'very satisfied'. Table 6 shows the patients' pretreatment and postcompletion responses to the four questions. It can be seen that three of these self-satisfaction measures improved from the earlier to the later time while the fourth, satisfaction with life in general remained the same. The only one of these measures to improve significantly, however, was satisfaction with opposite-sex relationships.

Interestingly, when questioned concerning their objective prior to the start of treatment, many of the patients mentioned wishing to be rid of taunting, staring, etc., but only one specified the wish to become more attractive to the opposite sex. Yet it appears that this result was, in the aggregate, obtained. Whether this outcome was largely unanticipated in advance or an important part of the hidden agenda all along can, at the present, be addressed only in speculation.

Broadly speaking, how do the patients feel about having taken part in the laser program? In the postcompletion survey, fully 93 percent of patients expressed some degree of satisfaction and only 7 percent indicated dissatisfaction with the effects of treatment on their lives. By the long-term follow-up, the percentage satisfied declined somewhat to 66 percent, with 16 percent dissatisfied and 17 percent neutral. In the dropout follow-up the satisfaction rate was, predictably, lower, with 47 percent satisfied in some degree and 53 percent dissatisfied. Since the primary factor we have identified as leading to dropping out is unfavorable physical results, the importance of being able to screen out those unlikely to be helped is underlined. However, many patients who were less than ecstatic about the treatment's effects still felt the program had been worth a try. One quite representative patient wrote that he felt 'satisfaction in knowing I did the most I could. ... It is better to undertake a treatment like this rather than end up 20 years from now getting angry with yourself (for not having taken the chance)'. In various ways this opinion was echoed among other patients. For example, when asked for advice to prospective patients, 85 percent of completion patients who responded counseled them to go ahead with treatment, as opposed to 15 percent who suggested holding off. Even among the dropout patients, more than twice as many advised prospective patients to go ahead with treatment as advised to avoid it.

To be sure, several of the patients, mainly among the dropouts, evaluated the treatment program with a terse statement to the effect that 'it was a waste of time'. A greater number were unrestrained in their praise. One woman, for example, wrote: 'The laser treatments have been the biggest positive changes I've ever gone through in my life. ... I feel certain that I'll continue to change and grow as a result of the treatments. Every part of my life will be touched and enriched'. A response perhaps closer to the center of our sample was offered by a young man (single at the start of treatment, now married) who wrote: 'My birthmark is still visible, but much less obvious than before the treatment. ... In some places where one treatment area meets another I think there are lines that were missed. These are not objectionable. ... Children no longer ask questions, women look longer. I'm satisfied.'

References

1. Kalick, S. M., Goldwyn, R. M., Noe, J. M. Social issues and body image concerns of port wine stain patients undergoing laser therapy. *Lasers in Surgery and Medicine.* 1981; **1**:205–13.
2. Noe, J. M., Barsky, S. H., Geer, D. E., *et al.* Port wine stains and the response to argon laser therapy: successful treatment and the predictive role of color, age, and biopsy. *Plast. Reconstr. Surg.* 1980; **65**:130–6.
3. Barsky, S. H., Rosen, S., Geer, D. E., *et al.* The nature and evolution of port wine stains: a computer-assisted study. *J. Invest. Dermatol.* 1980; **74**:154–7.
4. Larrow, L., Noe, J. M. Care of the patient with a port wine hemangioma. *Am. J. Nurs.* 1982; **82–5**:278–283.
5. Eysenck, H. J., Eysenck, S. B. G. *Manual for the Eysenck Personality Inventory.* San Diego: Educational and Industrial Testing Service, 1968.
6. Zuckerman, M., Lubin, B. *Manual for the Multiple Affect Adjective Checklist.* San Diego: Educational and Industrial Testing Service, 1965.
7. Spielberger, C. D., Gorsuch, R. L., Lushene, R. E. *STAI manual.* Palo Alto, California: Consulting Psychologists Press, 1970.

8. Robinson J., Shaver, P. *Measures of Social Psychological Attitudes*. Ann Arbor, Michigan: Institute for Social Research, 1973:84–7.
9. Edgerton, M. T., Jacobson, W. E., Meyer, E. Surgical-psychiatric study of patients seeking plastic (cosmetic) surgery: ninety-eight consecutive patients with minimal deformity. *Br. J. Plast. Surg.* 1961; **13**:136–45.
10. Reich, J. The surgery of appearance: psychological and related aspects. *Med. J. Aust.* 1969; **2**:5–13.
11. Goin, M. K., Burgoyne, R. W., Goin, J. M., *et al.* A prospective psychological study of 50 female face-life patients. *Plast Reconstr Surg.* 1980; **65**:436–42.
12. Goin, J. M., Goin, M. K. *Changing the Body: Psychological Effects of Plastic Surgery*. Baltimore: Williams & Wilkins, 1981.
13. Jacobson, W. E., Edgerton M. T., Meyer, E., *et al.* Psychiatric evaluation of male patients seeking cosmetic surgery. *Plast. Reconstr. Surg.* 1960; **26**:356–572.
14. Cousins, N. *Anatomy of an Illness as Perceived by the Patient*. New York: Norton, 1979.
15. Goldwyn, R. M. *The Patient and the Plastic Surgeon*. Boston: Little, Brown, 1981.
16. Macgregor, F. C. Personal communication. Also see Macgregor, F. C. *Transformation and Identify*. New York: New York Times Book Co., 1974, and Macgregor, F. C. *After Plastic Surgery*. New York: Praeger, 1979.

The Future of Lasers in Medicine

Cutaneous Lasery Therapy: Principles and Methods
Edited by K. A. Arndt, J. M. Noe, and S. Rosen
© 1983 John Wiley & Sons Ltd

21

Future Considerations of Lasers in Medicine

Leon Goldman

There is increasing interest in cutaneous laser therapy. With progress in laser surgery and medicine and in laser technology itself, there will continue to be a number of developments that will affect the use of the laser on the skin.

New lasers may be developed for therapy and there will be modifications of the instrumentation currently available in order to increase flexibility and to decrease costs. This is evident now with the 720 Sharplan CO_2 office laser model and with the use of reflection spectrophotometry on the surface of port wine stain (PWS) lesions. There will also be research and development on the waveguide Radio Frequency Excited CO_2 Laser for minor skin surgery. Increasing use of fiberoptic transmission, especially with thallium halide and zinc selenide, with the CO_2 laser will allow greater use in body cavities and for intralesional impacts. There will be interest in development of instrumentation for the oral cavity and the vaginal vault. Extension of instrumentation for microsurgery on vascular channels will allow use of intravascular fiberoptics for the direct induction of thrombogenesis and even for thrombolysis. These experiments will be of interst to those working on laser Doppler techniques for the treatment of strokes and for the canalization of occluded coronary vessels. We are developing intralesional fiberoptic probes for impacts on perivascular tissues.

Another exciting instrument will be the multiple-laser operating probe containing CO_2, argon, and Nd:YAG lasers in the same terminator. Although this apparatus will be most helpful to the cancer surgeon, thoracic surgeon, and neurosurgeon, it may also be of interest in skin surgery in the treatment of large, vascular lesions, metastatic skin cancers, large skin malignancies, and other lesions such as extensive disabling warts. Other technical modifications will include research and development to extend super pulses, such as with the Q-switched ruby lasers, to allow selective thermocoagulation necrosis with minimal effect on heating of adjacent structures. This will have value in laser surgery of vascular tumors as well as in plastic surgery, particularly on the face and neck. At the present time we are studying combined laser treatment of the 'thick lip' associated with the combined PWS and intraoral cavernous angioma. The argon laser is used on the skin and the CO_2 laser is used for extensive excisions of the oral cavity.

There will be increasing use of laser microsurgery for treatment of early neoplasms that have become evident by surface microscopy examination. This has been accomplished not only in animal experiments but in gynecologic surgery with the use of the colposcope. In this instance, the abnormal vascular pattern in the mucosal area may be seen very clearly, and the rapid destruction of the intrapithelial neoplasms by lasers is then easily carried out.

Extending the use of the ultraviolet laser will be dependent upon extensive studies on normal and abnormal vasculature of skin and mucous membranes. The preliminary experiments with this laser for the treatment of malignancies will also need to have more controlled experiments. Lasers may also serve as an adjunct in the rapidly developing field of cancer hyperthermia [1]. This may be combined with microwaves plus colloidal ion particles, as we have done, plus lasers in the visible light range transmitted even to metastatic lesions by fiberoptic transmission. Magnets may hold the colloidal ion particles to the metastatic area, if desired. The whole field of magnetobiology can be applied to laser cancer surgery. For additional studies on cancer hyperthermia, Radio Frequency (RF) localized treatment such as is being done now in the hyperthermia treatment of breast cancer, may be combined with laser surgery [2].

There will continue to be increasing development in laser-induced fluorescence for diagnosis and treatment of neoplastic lesions. This will be extended in the field of laser surgery, especially as regards skin malignancies. The search for fluorochromes other than hematoporphyrin derivatives and acridine orange which will be absorbed chiefly by abnormal mitotic tissue, and the use of local injection and implantation techniques, possibly even tattooing with these fluorochromes, may help to prevent photosensitizing reactions on uninvolved skin. For gastric malignancy, some of the cancer chemotherapeutic agents also show laser-induced fluorescence. This makes for a double strike against often inoperable gastric carcinoma. Such techniques may be applicable to massive inoperable skin carcinomas.

With the argon laser treatment of PWS, it is important that interest be shown in prevention of hypertrophic scar formation, especially of the lip and chin. At present we are using a plastic prosthesis for pressure lesions in these areas. This is applied shortly after treatment as an attempt at scar prevention. These prostheses were developed at the Shriners Burns Institute of the College of Medicine of the University of Cincinnati. It is evident that considerable research and controlled studies are necessary before lasers can be used to treat hypertrophic scarring. Our current studies in this area include not only tissue culture work but the treatment of hypertrophic scars in burn patients. The laser treatment of telangiectasia of the thigh and lower leg, especially in women, continues to offer a real challenge, since the results of such treatments are much less favorable than on the face, for unknown reasons. Such factors as stasis, incompetent valves, and increased venous pressures are often mentioned. Detailed basic studies are needed.

Especially important now is the factor of rebound telangiectasia around laser-treated area on the lower extremities. The interest of laser surgeons in the field of vascular dynamics in these sites is essential in order to understand and control laser treatment of these vascular problems. We are using special intravascular fiberoptic transmission probes which we have developed, as mentioned previously.

The so-called areas of biostimulation must be studied and clarified, and controls must definitely be used. I refer not only to graft replacement procedures where the recipient area is stimulated by low-output laser radiation, but also to the healing of chronic infections and the healing of ulcers. The effect of lasers on T and B cells and the entire new field of laser immunology including the development of monoclonal antibodies must be expanded.

It has to be emphasized that one cannot have progress in any phase of laser medicine without basic work on laser biology. Such studies must include not only those on microirradiation, laser biophysics, chemistry, laser spectroscopy, acoustical holography, and the development of protocols for photoreactions in tissue, but also for safety programs for any new laser systems that may be introduced for phototherapy.

Finally, we have to teach cutaneous laser therapy. We must take trained dermatologists or plastic surgeons and then instruct them in laser and medical technology. The new revolutions in laser communications and laser information handling may serve as a very effective visual aid in such training. The hope of the future is the attempt to develop three-dimensional imagery in laser communication programs in order to allow better teaching in fields such as dermatology and plastic surgery. The ambulatory surgical center [3] offers great opportunity for the development of laser surgery with easy availability of expensive current laser surgical instruments, various types of anesthesia, and expert help and consultation from colleagues in other disciplines.

The dream of laser medicine of the future includes also laser perinatology [4] extending from laser microsurgery on chromosomes to the newborn infant. Along with current developments on laser scanning of karyotypes it has become possible to alter specific areas of chromosomes by microirradiation. With the combination of acoustical holography with lasers, visualization of the fetus *in utero* is possible. With the laser microprobe it may be possible to take tissue for spectroscopic analysis and mosaicism and perform surgery for polydactyly and perhaps even on early progressive angiomas. After birth, there may be early laser surgery of congenital abnormalities.

There is much in the future for lasers in medicine and biology to stimulate and challenge us all.

References

1. Goldman, I. (ed.) *The Biomedical Laser. Technology and Clinical Applications.* New York: Springer-Verlag, 1981:325.
2. Goldman, L., Dreffer, R., Microwaves, magnetic ion particles and lasers as a combined test model for investigations of hyperthermia treatment of cancer. *Arch. Dermatol. Res.* 1976; **257**:227–8.
3. Goldman, L. Dermatologic surgery in an ambulatory surgical center: 10 years experience. In press.
4. Goldman, L., Reed, K. Laser—some investigative procedure in perinatology. *Acta Medicotechnica.* 1982; **30**:15–16.

Index

237